T0260429

Current Classification of Vascular Anomalies (2013)

TUMORS	Slow-Flow
Infantile Hemangioma PHACES association LUMBAR association	**Capillary Malformation** CLAPO Cutis marmorata Cutis marmorata telangiectatica congenita Diffuse capillary malformation with overgrowth Fading capillary stain Heterotopic neural nodule Macrocephaly–capillary malformation
Congenital Hemangioma Rapidly involuting Noninvoluting	**Lymphatic Malformation** Macrocystic Microcystic Combined (macrocystic/microcystic) Primary lymphedema Gorham-Stout disease Generalized lymphatic anomaly Kaposiform lymphangiomatosis
Kaposiform Hemangioendothelioma	**Venous Malformation** Blue rubber bleb nevus syndrome Cerebral cavernous malformation Cutaneomucosal venous malformation Diffuse phlebectasia of Bockenheimer Fibroadipose vascular anomaly Glomuvenous malformation Phlebectasia Sinus pericranii Verrucous venous malformation
Pyogenic Granuloma	
Rare Vascular Tumors Angiosarcoma Cutaneovisceral angiomatosis with thrombocytopenia Enzinger intramuscular hemangioma Epithelioid hemangioendothelioma Infantile myofibroma Tufted angioma	

MALFORMATIONS

Fast-Flow	Overgrowth Syndromes
Arteriovenous Malformation	CLOVES
Capillary malformation–arteriovenous malformation	Klippel-Trenaunay
Hereditary hemorrhagic telangiectasia	Maffucci
PTEN-associated vascular anomaly	Parkes Weber
Wyburn-Mason syndrome	Proteus
	Sturge-Weber

KEY

CLAPO, Acronym for *c*apillary malformation of the *l*ower lip, *l*ymphatic malformation of the face and neck, *a*symmetry of face and limbs, and *p*artial or generalized *o*vergrowth; *CLOVES,* Acronym for *c*ongenital, *l*ipomatous, *o*vergrowth, *v*ascular malformations, *e*pidermal nevi, and *s*pinal/skeletal anomalies and/or scoliosis; *LUMBAR,* Acronym for *l*ower body hemangioma and other cutaneous defects, *u*rogenital anomalies, ulceration, *m*yelopathy, *b*ony deformities, *a*norectal malformations, arterial anomalies, and *r*enal anomalies syndrome; *PHACES,* Acronym for *p*osterior fossa brain malformation, *h*emangioma, *a*rterial cerebrovascular anomalies, *c*oarctation of the aorta and cardiac defects, *e*ye/endocrine abnormalities, *s*ternal clefting/supraumbilical raphe; *PTEN,* phosphatase and tensin homolog gene.

Vascular Anomalies
Classification, Diagnosis, & Management

VASCULAR ANOMALIES
Classification, Diagnosis, & Management

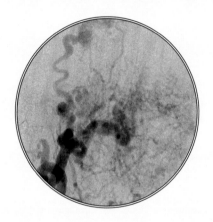

Arin K. Greene, MD, MMSc
Department of Plastic and Oral Surgery,
Vascular Anomalies Center, Boston Children's Hospital;
Associate Professor of Surgery, Harvard Medical School,
Boston, Massachusetts

Quality Medical Publishing, Inc.
St. Louis, Missouri
2013

PUBLISHER Karen Berger
EDITORIAL DIRECTOR Michelle Berger
DIRECTOR OF EDITING Suzanne Wakefield
VICE PRESIDENT OF PRODUCTION AND MANUFACTURING Carolyn Reich
DIRECTOR OF GRAPHICS Brett Stone
GRAPHICS PRODUCTION Ngoc-Thuy Khuu
LAYOUT ARTIST Carol Hollett
COVER DESIGN Amanda Tomasikiewicz

Quality Medical Publishing, Inc.
2248 Welsch Industrial Court
St. Louis, Missouri 63146
Telephone: 1-314-878-7808; 1-800-348-7808
Web site: *http://www.qmp.com*

LIBRARY OF CONGRESS CATALOGING-IN-PUBLICATION DATA

Greene, Arin K., author.
 Vascular anomalies : classification, diagnosis, & management / Arin K. Greene.
    p. ; cm.
  Includes bibliographical references and index.
  ISBN 978-1-57626-399-0 (pbk.)
  I. Title.
  [DNLM: 1. Vascular Malformations--diagnosis. 2. Vascular Malformations--therapy. WG 220]
  RC388.5
  616.8'1--dc23
                          2013013999

QM/F/F
5   4   3   2   1

This book is dedicated to patients with vascular anomalies—
I hope it translates into improved therapies

PREFACE

Vascular anomalies affect at least 5% of the population and can cause significant morbidity. The etiopathogenesis of vascular anomalies remains poorly understood, and many treatments are unsatisfactory. Because vascular anomalies can affect any area of the body, most medical and surgical specialists manage patients with these lesions. The field can be intimidating, because numerous types of vascular anomalies exist, different vascular anomalies often look similar, and the terminology used to describe these lesions has been confusing. The goal of this book is to provide an easy-to-use reference to facilitate the treatment of patients with vascular anomalies.

Arterial malformations, such as aneurysm, atresia, ectasia, and stenosis, are not presented here, because these anomalies are rarely seen in a vascular anomalies center; they are primarily managed by an interventional radiologist, cardiologist, or vascular/cardiac surgeon. Noneponymous combined vascular malformations, such as lymphatic-venous malformation, have not been separated from the major types of vascular malformations because they are managed similarly, based on the problematic component of the lesion. A chapter is dedicated to primary lymphedema because the disease is significantly different from other types of lymphatic malformations. A recurring feature is a table that provides the current classifications of vascular anomalies.

Vascular Anomalies: Classification, Diagnosis, & Management was designed to be portable so that it can be carried by the health care provider for quick reference when treating a patient with a vascular anomaly. The text is clinically oriented, rather than focusing on history or research. Clinical features, etiopathogenesis, differential diagnosis, appropriate imaging studies, and operative and nonoperative management are presented for each anomaly.

The book can also be used as a source of information for more in-depth study of the subject, teaching, or research. I hope this text will stimulate readers to improve our understanding of these lesions and to develop better treatments.

Arin K. Greene

ACKNOWLEDGMENTS

During my childhood I aspired to become a pediatric plastic surgeon because my youngest brother was born with a cleft lip and palate. I witnessed the problems he experienced because of his facial deformity, and how it affected him and the rest of our family.

As a medical student, I traveled from Chicago to Boston to visit John Mulliken because of his international reputation as a cleft surgeon. While in his clinic, I was introduced to patients with vascular anomalies and felt that many of the children had significantly worse problems than my brother's cleft lip and palate. I was troubled by the significant morbidity that vascular anomalies could cause, the lack of understanding regarding their etiopathogenesis, and the often less than satisfactory treatments. As Dr. Mulliken would say, I developed a "sense of wonder" for the field of vascular anomalies and became focused on improving the lives of these patients.

Like all physicians, I have been molded by my mentors. I want to thank John Mulliken, who trained me in the field of vascular anomalies, and who has had the greatest influence on my career. I am also extremely grateful to Steven Fishman, who has been a mentor in the field of vascular anomalies; Judah Folkman, who taught me vascular biology and how to become a surgeon-scientist; Robert Goldwyn, who mentored me during my general surgery training; James May, who was my most influential teacher during my plastic surgery residency; John Meara, who has given me tremendous professional support; and Sumner Slavin, who stimulated my interest in the field of lymphedema.

I would like to thank Karen Berger and the team at Quality Medical Publishing for their outstanding work in putting this book together. Many individuals at QMP contributed to the project: Andrew Berger, Michelle Berger, Carol Hollett, Thuy Khuu, Carolyn Reich, Brett Stone, and Suzanne Wakefield. I am privileged to be a part of the QMP "family" that has produced so many important texts in the field of plastic and reconstructive surgery.

Finally, I want to acknowledge my family for their support. I am not sure I would be a plastic surgeon today without my grandparents, Albert and Ruth, who had a profound influence on my life. And foremost, I want to thank my wife, Sarah, and three boys, Albert, Mac, and Henry, who encourage and support the passion I have for my "job."

CONTENTS

VASCULAR ANOMALIES
Classification, Diagnosis, & Management

I

The Field of
Vascular Anomalies

CHAPTER 1

Introduction

BACKGROUND

- Vascular anomalies are disorders of the endothelium that can affect capillaries, arteries, veins, or lymphatics.
- Any anatomic structure can be involved; thus most medical specialties manage patients with these lesions.
- Vascular anomalies are relatively common, affecting approximately 5.5% of the population.
- Lesions are usually diagnosed during infancy or childhood, although they can rarely present in adulthood.
- The field is confusing, because numerous types of vascular anomalies exist, different lesions often look similar, and many practitioners use imprecise terminology (Fig. 1-1).

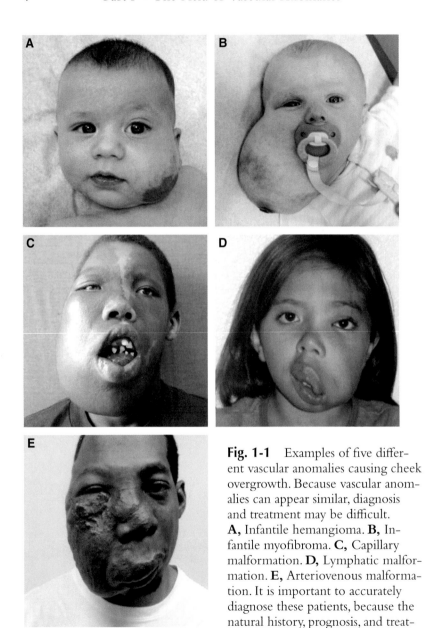

Fig. 1-1   Examples of five different vascular anomalies causing cheek overgrowth. Because vascular anomalies can appear similar, diagnosis and treatment may be difficult. **A,** Infantile hemangioma. **B,** Infantile myofibroma. **C,** Capillary malformation. **D,** Lymphatic malformation. **E,** Arteriovenous malformation. It is important to accurately diagnose these patients, because the natural history, prognosis, and treatment of each of the five cheek lesions are different.

MORBIDITY

- Vascular anomalies are almost always benign.
- Because lesions typically involve the integument, the most common problem they cause is disfigurement/psychosocial morbidity.
- Local complications consist of bleeding, destruction of anatomic structures, infection, obstruction, pain, thrombosis, and ulceration.
- Systemic morbidity can include congestive heart failure, disseminated intravascular coagulation (DIC), pulmonary embolism, thrombocytopenia, and sepsis.
- Many types of vascular anomalies are progressive, recur following treatment, and cannot be cured.

MANAGEMENT

- Because vascular anomalies usually involve the skin and present during childhood, patients often are initially referred to a pediatric plastic surgeon or pediatric dermatologist.
- Many lesions cannot be cured, and thus pediatric patients may eventually be treated by adult physicians.
- Although certain types of vascular anomalies can be managed by a single physician with expertise in the field, many lesions require the care of multiple specialists.
- Often the goal of treatment is to control, rather than to cure, the vascular anomaly.
- Vascular anomalies centers now exist in many academic centers where patients can receive coordinated care by an interdisciplinary team of specialists.
- Patients with problematic vascular anomalies should be referred to an interdisciplinary vascular anomalies center. The field is complicated, and patients are more likely to be diagnosed and treated correctly when managed in a program specializing in these conditions.

- The most common specialties caring for patients with vascular anomalies include plastic surgery, dermatology, diagnostic/interventional radiology, hematology/oncology, general/pediatric surgery, orthopedic surgery, vascular surgery, ophthalmology, otolaryngology, cardiology, endocrinology, and neurosurgery.
- Despite improved treatments for vascular anomalies, many lesions continue to cause significant morbidity and are not curable.
- As the etiopathogenesis of vascular anomalies becomes better understood, prevention of these diseases may become possible.

CURRENT STATE OF THE FIELD

- Research in the field of vascular anomalies continues to improve.
- Basic studies have been limited by the lack of animal models that recapitulate human disease. In the future, animal models will provide insight into the etiopathogenesis of vascular anomalies and will enable the testing of novel therapies.
- Clinical investigation has been handicapped, particularly for vascular malformations, by the (1) use of incorrect terminology in the literature, (2) heterogeneity of the lesions (for example, one lymphatic malformation may be small and located on an extremity, while another could involve the entire face), and (3) lack of large databases of patients with these relatively rare conditions.
- Clinical research will be facilitated as the number of patients being treated in well-organized centers continues to increase. In addition, new vascular anomalies will be identified as data on larger numbers of patients with rare lesions are collected.
- Several of these disorders continue to cause significant morbidity, and their etiopathogenesis remains poorly understood.

- Vascular malformations generally are more problematic than vascular tumors and are more likely to require interdisciplinary care. Drugs are available to treat tumors, whereas standard systemic pharmacotherapy is not available to treat malformations. Two thirds of patients referred to our Vascular Anomalies Center have a vascular malformation, although these are 10 times less common than vascular tumors.

Selected References

Greene AK. Current concepts of vascular anomalies. J Craniofac Surg 23:220-224, 2012.

Greene AK. Vascular anomalies: current overview of the field. Clin Plast Surg 38:1-5, 2011.

Greene AK, Liu AS, Mulliken JB, Chalache K, Fishman SJ. Vascular anomalies in 5621 patients: guidelines for referral. J Pediatr Surg 46:1784-1789, 2011.

Hassanein A, Mulliken JB, Fishman SJ, Greene AK. Evaluation of terminology for vascular anomalies in current literature. Plast Reconstr Surg 127:347-351, 2011.

CHAPTER 2

Classification and Terminology

CLASSIFICATION

• Vascular anomalies are classified biologically, based on their clinical behavior and cellular characteristics. This system was proposed by Mulliken and Glowacki in 1982 (Table 2-1) and adopted by the International Society for the Study of Vascular Anomalies (ISSVA) in 1996 (Table 2-2).

Table 2-1	*Biological Classification of Vascular Lesions in Infants and Children (1982)*	
HEMANGIOMAS	**MALFORMATIONS**	
Proliferating phase	Capillary	
Involuting phase	Venous	
	Arterial	
	Lymphatic	
	Fistulas	

From Mulliken JB, Glowacki J. Hemangiomas and vascular malformations in infants and children: a classification based on endothelial characteristics. Plast Reconstr Surg 69:412-422, 1982.

9

Table 2-2 *International Society for the Study of Vascular Anomalies Classification of Vascular Anomalies (1996)*

TUMORS	MALFORMATIONS	
	Simple	**Combined**
Hemangioma	Capillary	AVF, AVM, CVM, CLVM
	Lymphatic	LVM, CAVM, CLAVM
Other	Venous	
	Arterial	

From Enjolras O, Mulliken JB. Vascular tumors and vascular malformations (new issues). Adv Dermatol 13:375-423, 1997.

AVF, Arteriovenous fistula; *AVM*, arteriovenous malformation; *CAVM*, capillary-arteriovenous malformation; *CLAVM*, capillary-lymphatic-arteriovenous malformation; *CLVM*, capillary-lymphatic-venous malformation; *CVM*, capillary-venous malformation; *LVM*, lymphatic-venous malformation.

- Using the biologic classification of vascular anomalies, 90% or more of lesions can be diagnosed by history and physical examination.
- There are two broad types of vascular anomalies: tumors and malformations.
  - Tumors demonstrate endothelial proliferation and are more common than malformations. They affect approximately 5% of the population. There are four major types: infantile hemangioma, congenital hemangioma, kaposiform hemangioendothelioma, and pyogenic granuloma (Fig. 2-1).
  - Vascular malformations are errors in vascular development and have stable endothelial turnover. They affect approximately 0.5% of the population. There are four major categories based

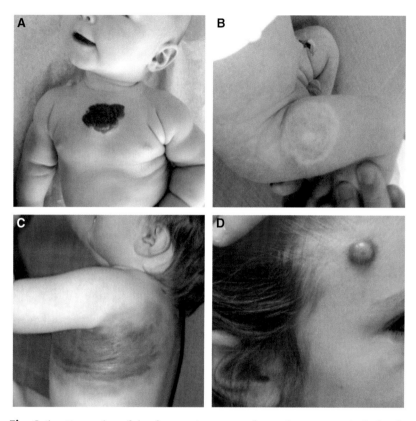

Fig. 2-1   Examples of the four major types of vascular tumors. **A,** Infantile hemangioma. **B,** Congenital hemangioma. **C,** Kaposiform hemangioendothelioma. **D,** Pyogenic granuloma.

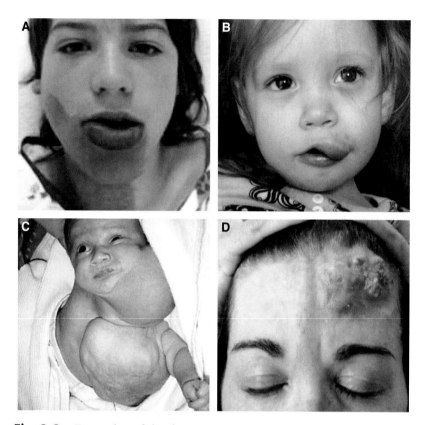

Fig. 2-2 Examples of the four major types of vascular malformations. **A,** Capillary malformation. **B,** Venous malformation. **C,** Lymphatic malformation. **D,** Arteriovenous malformation.

  on the primary vessel that is malformed: capillary malformation, lymphatic malformation, venous malformation, and arteriovenous malformation (Fig. 2-2).
  – Malformations are further divided into rheologically slow-
    flow lesions (capillary, lymphatic, venous) and fast-flow le-
    sions (arteriovenous malformation, arterial aneurysm/atresia/
    ectasia/stenosis).
- There are many phenotypic subtypes of the major categories of
  vascular anomalies (for example, glomuvenous malformation),
  combined lesions (capillary-lymphatic-venous malformation),
  and eponymous syndromes (Parkes Weber syndrome).
- The classification of vascular anomalies continues to expand and
  become more precise as our knowledge of these lesions evolves
  (Table 2-3). For example, congenital hemangiomas and kaposiform hemangioendotheliomas have been differentiated from infantile hemangiomas. Genetic studies have identified subtypes of
  venous malformations, such as cutaneomucosal and glomuvenous.
  New vascular anomalies, such as the PTEN-associated vascular
  anomaly, and syndromes (congenital, lipomatous, overgrowth,
  vascular malformations, epidermal nevi and spinal/skeletal
  anomalies and/or scoliosis [CLOVES] syndrome) continue to be
  characterized.
- Despite the widening classification of vascular anomalies, 5% of
  patients referred to our center are still unable to be diagnosed
  and have vascular anomalies that have not yet been defined.

Table 2-3 Current Classification of Vascular Anomalies (2013)

TUMORS	Slow-Flow
Infantile Hemangioma PHACES association LUMBAR association	**Capillary Malformation** CLAPO Cutis marmorata Cutis marmorata telangiectatica congeni Diffuse capillary malformation with overgrowth Fading capillary stain Heterotopic neural nodule Macrocephaly–capillary malformation
Congenital Hemangioma Rapidly involuting Noninvoluting	**Lymphatic Malformation** Macrocystic Microcystic Combined (macrocystic/microcystic) Primary lymphedema Gorham-Stout disease Generalized lymphatic anomaly Kaposiform lymphangiomatosis
Kaposiform **Hemangioendothelioma**	**Venous Malformation** Blue rubber bleb nevus syndrome Cerebral cavernous malformation Cutaneomucosal venous malformation Diffuse phlebectasia of Bockenheimer Fibroadipose vascular anomaly Glomuvenous malformation Phlebectasia Sinus pericranii Verrucous venous malformation
Pyogenic Granuloma	
Rare Vascular Tumors Angiosarcoma Cutaneovisceral angiomatosis with thrombocytopenia Enzinger intramuscular hemangioma Epithelioid hemangioendothelioma Infantile myofibroma Tufted angioma	

MALFORMATIONS

Fast-Flow	Overgrowth Syndromes
Arterial Malformation Aneurysm Atresia Ectasia Stenosis	CLOVES Klippel-Trenaunay Maffucci Parkes Weber Proteus Sturge-Weber
Arteriovenous Malformation Capillary malformation–arteriovenous malformation Hereditary hemorrhagic telangiectasia *PTEN*-associated vascular anomaly Wyburn-Mason syndrome	

KEY

CLAPO, Acronym for *c*apillary malformation of the lower *l*ip, *l*ymphatic malformation of the face and neck, *a*symmetry of face and limbs, and *p*artial or generalized *o*vergrowth; *CLOVES,* Acronym for *c*ongenital, *l*ipomatous, *o*vergrowth, *v*ascular malformations, *e*pidermal nevi, and *s*pinal/skeletal anomalies and/or scoliosis; *LUMBAR,* Acronym for *l*ower body hemangioma and other cutaneous defects, *u*rogenital anomalies, ulceration, *m*yelopathy, *b*ony deformities, *a*norectal malformations, arterial anomalies, and *r*enal anomalies syndrome; *PHACES,* Acronym for *p*osterior fossa brain malformation, *h*emangioma, *a*rterial cerebrovascular anomalies, *c*oarctation of the aorta and cardiac defects, *e*ye/endocrine abnormalities, *s*ternal clefting/supraumbilical raphe; *PTEN,* phosphatase and tensin homolog gene.

TERMINOLOGY

- The field of vascular anomalies has been impeded by imprecise terminology, which has created diagnostic confusion, blocked communication between physicians, inhibited research, and caused incorrect treatment.
- Historically, vascular anomalies were labeled descriptively according to the type of food they resembled ("cherry," "strawberry," "port-wine"). They were later divided histopathologically into *angioma simplex* (superficial hemangioma), *angioma cavernosum* (deep hemangioma/venous malformation), or *angioma racemosum* (arteriovenous malformation). Lymphatic malformation was separated into *lymphangioma* and *cystic hygroma*.
- Capillary or strawberry hemangioma became associated with a hemangioma affecting the dermis, which appears red. Hemangioma located below the skin is bluish and was often called *cavernous hemangioma*. The terms *capillary* and *cavernous* were also used to describe capillary malformation and venous malformation, respectively. Another label for capillary malformation was *port-wine stain*. Cystic hygroma and lymphangioma became common terms for macrocystic lymphatic malformation and microcystic lymphatic malformation, respectively. Hemangioma continued to be used to describe any type of vascular anomaly, including both tumors and malformations.
- Terminology was clarified using the biologic classification of vascular anomalies because the suffix -oma, meaning upregulated cellular growth, was reserved for vascular tumors. Thus terms such as lymphangioma (microcystic lymphatic malformation), cystic hygroma (macrocystic lymphatic malformation), and cavernous hemangioma (venous malformation), which describe nonproliferating malformations, were no longer used.
- Although significant progress has been made, incorrect terminology continues to pervade the medical community, and it remains difficult to conduct clinical research and communicate with other physicians. For example, 47% of patients evaluated in our center have an incorrect referral diagnosis; malformations

are more likely to be misdiagnosed (54%) compared with tumors (30%).

- The use of imprecise terminology also increases the likelihood that a patient will be treated incorrectly. In a review of the 2009 literature with manuscripts containing the term hemangioma, 71% of authors used hemangioma erroneously to describe another vascular anomaly. Patients whose lesions were mislabeled were more likely to be managed incorrectly (21%), compared with patients whose anomalies were correctly designated using standardized International Society for the Study of Vascular Anomalies (ISSVA) terminology (0.0%) ($p < 0.0001$).

- Continuing education is essential to increase the use of accepted biologic terms for vascular anomalies (Table 2-4).

Table 2-4 *Incorrect Terminology Used to Describe Vascular Anomalies*

TUMORS		MALFORMATIONS	
Biologic Name	**Incorrect Term**	**Biologic Name**	**Incorrect Term**
Infantile hemangioma	Capillary hemangioma Cavernous hemangioma Strawberry hemangioma	Capillary malformation	Port-wine stain Capillary hemangioma
Kaposiform hemangio-endothelioma	Capillary hemangioma	Lymphatic malformation	Cystic hygroma Lymphangioma
Pyogenic granuloma	Hemangioma	Venous malformation	Cavernous hemangioma
		Arteriovenous malformation	Arteriovenous hemangioma

Selected References

Enjolras O, Mulliken JB. Vascular tumors and vascular malformations (new issues). Adv Dermatol 13:375-423, 1997.

Finn MC, Glowacki J, Mulliken JB. Congenital vascular lesions: clinical application of a new classification. J Pediatr Surg 18:894-900, 1983.

Greene AK. Vascular anomalies: current overview of the field. Clin Plast Surg 38:1-5, 2011.

Greene AK, Liu AS, Mulliken JB, Chalache K, Fishman SJ. Vascular anomalies in 5621 patients: guidelines for referral. J Pediatr Surg 46:1784-1789, 2011.

Hassanein A, Mulliken JB, Fishman SJ, Greene AK. Evaluation of terminology for vascular anomalies in current literature. Plast Reconstr Surg 127:347-351, 2011.

Meyer JS, Hoffer FA, Barnes PD, Mulliken JB. Biological classification of soft-tissue vascular anomalies: MR correlation. AJR Am J Roentgenol 157:559-564, 1991.

Mulliken JB, Glowacki J. Hemangiomas and vascular malformations in infants and children: a classification based on endothelial characteristics. Plast Reconstr Surg 69:412-422, 1982.

Vascular Tumors

II

TUMORS	MALFORMATIONS		
	Slow-Flow	**Fast-Flow**	**Overgrowth Syndromes**
Infantile Hemangioma PHACES association LUMBAR association	*Capillary Malformation*	*Arteriovenous Malformation*	CLOVES Klippel-Trenaunay Maffucci Parkes Weber Proteus Sturge-Weber
Congenital Hemangioma Rapidly involuting Noninvoluting	*Lymphatic Malformation*		
Kaposiform Hemangioendothelioma	*Venous Malformation*		
Pyogenic Granuloma			

Rare Vascular Tumors
Angiosarcoma
Cutaneovisceral angiomatosis
  with thrombocytopenia
Enzinger intramuscular
  hemangioma
Epithelioid hemangioendo-
  thelioma
Infantile myofibroma
Tufted angioma			

CHAPTER [3]

Infantile Hemangioma

TUMORS	MALFORMATIONS		
	Slow-Flow	**Fast-Flow**	**Overgrowth Syndromes**
Infantile Hemangioma PHACES association LUMBAR association	*Capillary Malformation*	*Arteriovenous Malformation*	CLOVES Klippel-Trenaunay Maffucci Parkes Weber Proteus Sturge-Weber
Congenital Hemangioma	*Lymphatic Malformation*		
Kaposiform Hemangioendothelioma	*Venous Malformation*		
Pyogenic Granuloma			
Rare Vascular Tumors			

CLINICAL FEATURES

- Infantile hemangioma (IH) is a benign neoplasm of the endothelium.
- It is the most common tumor of infancy, affecting 4% to 5% of white individuals.
- Its prevalence is inversely related to skin color (that is, the darker the skin color, the lower the risk).
- Females (4:1) are affected more frequently than males.
- Children born prematurely are more likely to develop an infantile hemangioma. The risk is increased 40% for every 500 g decrease in birth weight less than 2500 g.
- 80% involve the integument and appear bright red (*superficial* infantile hemangioma).
- 20% are underneath the skin and may appear bluish or have no overlying skin discoloration (*deep* infantile hemangioma).
- Infantile hemangioma is usually single (80%) and affects the head and neck (60%), trunk (25%), or extremity (15%).
- 50% are noted at birth by a telangiectatic stain/ecchymotic area, although the median age at presentation is 2 weeks after birth.
- During the first 9 months of life, infantile hemangioma grows rapidly *(proliferating phase);* 80% of its size is achieved by the time the infant is 3.2 ($\pm$ 1.7) months of age (Fig. 3-1).
- Between 9 and 12 months of age, the lesion begins to slowly shrink *(involuting phase);* the color fades and the lesion flattens. The appearance improves until 3½ years of age.
- After 3½ years of age, an infantile hemangioma will no longer be visible in 50% of children. Others will have a permanent deformity: residual telangiectasias, anetoderma from loss of elastic fibers, scarring, fibrofatty residuum, redundant skin, and/or destroyed anatomic structures.
- All infantile hemangiomas express type 3 iodothyronine deiodinase that deactivates thyroid hormone. However, only multifocal (21%) or diffuse (100%) hepatic lesions express enough of the deiodinase to cause hypothyroidism (although it is possible that a very large cutaneous lesion could cause hypothyroidism as well).

- A diffuse, superficial infantile hemangioma in a "segmental" distribution can exhibit minimal postnatal growth and be associated with underlying structural anomalies (PHACES association, LUMBAR association).

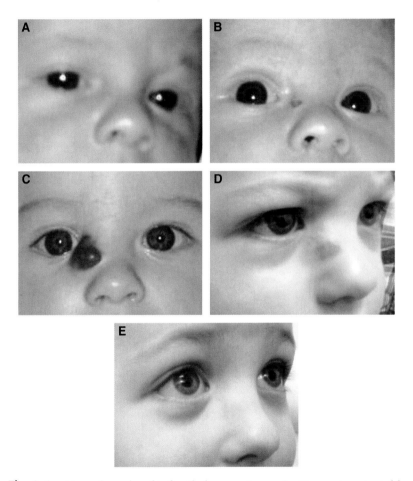

Fig. 3-1 Growth cycle of infantile hemangioma. **A,** Tumor is not visible at 2 weeks of age. **B,** Lesion is growing at 5 weeks of age. **C,** At 6 months the tumor is significantly larger. **D,** The tumor is involuting at 18 months of age. **E,** After involution, the infantile hemangioma is difficult to appreciate at 3½ years of age.

ETIOPATHOGENESIS

- Infantile hemangioma may arise from vasculogenesis (formation of blood vessels from progenitor cells).
- Hemangioma endothelial cells (HemECs) are clonal, and thus a somatic mutation in a precursor cell may cause the lesion. The life cycle of the tumor may be influenced extrinsically, by upregulated or downregulated local angiogenic factors.
- The precursor cell for infantile hemangioma might be a multipotent hemangioma-derived–stem cell (HemSC) that has been isolated. HemSCs produce human GLUT1-positive microvessels after clonal expansion in immunodeficient mice. Although it has been postulated that the precursor cell for infantile hemangioma may have embolized from the placenta, genetic studies have shown that HemECs are derived from the child, not the mother.
- Several mechanisms could contribute to the rapid growth of infantile hemangioma.
  - Hypoxia might stimulate circulating hemangioma-derived endothelial progenitor cell (HemEPC) recruitment to the tumor (increased circulating endothelial progenitor cells have been found in children with infantile hemangioma).
  - HemECs have been shown to have defective NFAT activity that decreases VEGFR-1 expression. Because VEGFR-1 acts as a decoy receptor, more VEFG-A becomes available to bind to VEGFR-2, which stimulates endothelial proliferation.
  - Local factors, such as a reduction in anti-angiogenic proteins, also may stimulate growth.
- The mechanism by which infantile hemangioma involutes is unknown.
  - As endothelial proliferation slows, apoptosis increases, and the lesion is replaced by fibrofatty tissue.
  - Apoptosis begins before 1 year of age and peaks at 24 months of age, causing a reduction in tumor volume.
  - Increased angiogenesis inhibitors in the epidermis overlying the hemangioma may promote involution.

— The source of adipocytes during involution is HemSCs, which also may differentiate into pericytes.

DIAGNOSIS

History and Physical Examination

- 90% or more of infantile hemangiomas are diagnosed by history and physical examination based on the tumor's appearance and unique growth cycle (Fig. 3-2).
- Deeper lesions are more difficult to diagnose, because they are noted later than superficial tumors and may not have significant overlying skin changes. A lesion beneath the integument might not be appreciated until 3 or 4 months of age, when it has grown large enough to cause a visible deformity.
- Diagnosis of deep or equivocal lesions is facilitated using a hand-held Doppler audio device, which shows fast-flow.

Imaging

- Ultrasonography is the first-line confirmatory study for a soft tissue infantile hemangioma if history, physical examination, and handheld Doppler findings are equivocal. Ultrasound is also used to identify hepatic lesions. Infantile hemangioma appears as a well-circumscribed hypervascular soft tissue mass. Low-resistance arterial waveforms indicate decreased arterial resistance and increased venous drainage.
- MRI is rarely indicated and requires sedation. It is necessary if a visceral lesion (for example, in the brain or lung) is suspected, or occasionally if the diagnosis remains unclear following ultrasonography.
  - During the proliferating phase, the MRI appearance of infantile hemangioma is a parenchymal mass with dilated feeding and draining vessels. Signal-voids represent fast-flow and shunting. The tumor is isointense on T1 sequences, hyper-

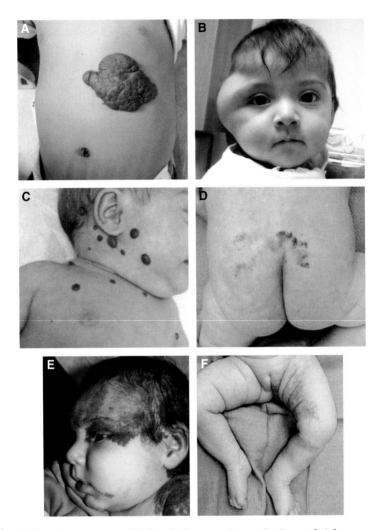

Fig. 3-2 Phenotypes of infantile hemangioma. **A,** Superficial tumor affecting primarily the integument. **B,** Deep lesion involving the subcutis. Note normal overlying skin color. **C,** Infant with multiple small cutaneous tumors (hemangiomatosis) as well as hepatic hemangioma. **D,** Patient with a superficial midline lesion overlying a lipomyelomeningocele. **E,** Infant with PHACE association. **F,** Neonate with LUMBAR reticular hemangioma affecting the lower extremity and perineum/genitalia.

intense on T2 images, and enhances homogeneously with contrast.
- An involuting infantile hemangioma on MRI shows increased lobularity and adipose tissue with areas of increased signal on T1 images. Lesions have reduced vessels, signal-voids, and contrast enhancement.

Histopathology

- Less than 1% of infantile hemangiomas require histopathology for diagnosis.
- Biopsy is obtained if a malignancy is suspected or the diagnosis remains equivocal following imaging studies.
- A proliferating infantile hemangioma shows tightly packed capillaries with plump endothelial cells (mitoses are present), thin basement membranes, and a layer of pericytes. Intervascular stroma is minimal, with few fibroblasts or mast cells.
- An involuting tumor has a reduced number of capillaries, enlargement of vascular channels, flattening of endothelium, apoptosis, reduced mitoses, and thickening of the basement membrane. Intervascular fibrous stroma and mast cells are increased.
- An involuted infantile hemangioma is primarily fibrofatty. The dermis can be scarred, with reduced elastic fibers and appendages. Few small residual capillaries are present that have thick basement membranes and often occluded lumens.
- An erythrocyte-type glucose transporter (GLUT1) is expressed in the endothelium of all growth phases of infantile hemangioma. Immunostaining for GLUT1 can differentiate infantile hemangioma from other vascular anomalies.

PHENOTYPIC CONSIDERATIONS

Head and Neck Location

- 10% of infantile hemangiomas cause significant problems during the proliferative phase, almost always when they are located on the head or neck.
- Scalp or eyebrow lesions may cause alopecia, because infantile hemangioma can damage hair follicles.
- Ulcerated tumors may destroy sensitive structures (for example, the eyelid, ear, nose, or lip).
- Obstruction of the external auditory canal can cause otitis externa, but sensorineural hearing loss does not occur if the contralateral canal is patent.
- Periorbital infantile hemangioma can block the visual axis, causing deprivation amblyopia, or distort the cornea, leading to astigmatic amblyopia. Infantile hemangioma of the upper eyelid is more likely to be problematic than a lesion involving the lower eyelid. Infants with periorbital tumors are referred to an ophthalmologist; the noninvolved orbit may be patched for 2 or more hours per day to stimulate use of the affected eye.
- Subglottic infantile hemangioma, which is associated with large cervicofacial lesions, may obstruct the airway. Patients are referred to an otolaryngologist for evaluation. The patency of the airway is usually maintained with oral pharmacotherapy; laser treatment or tracheostomy is rarely necessary.

Multiple Lesions

- Infants with five or more small (5 mm or less), domelike cutaneous infantile hemangiomas (hemangiomatosis) have a 16% risk for visceral lesions.
- The liver (usually multifocal) is most commonly affected (92% are asymptomatic). The brain, intestines, and lungs are rarely involved.
- Ultrasonography is used to rule out hepatic hemangiomas, although imaging is not mandatory, because intervention is not

required for an incidentally found lesion. Infants with problematic hepatic hemangiomas are usually symptomatic (for example, jaundice or failure to thrive) before they are referred for evaluation of the cutaneous lesions.

- If symptomatic brain, gastrointestinal, or lung lesions are suspected, an MRI is obtained.

Hepatic Location

- The liver is the most common extracutaneous site for hemangioma. There are three types: focal (28%), multifocal (57%), and diffuse (15%).
- *Focal hepatic hemangioma* is a rapidly involuting congenital hemangioma (RICH) that regresses immediately after birth. Males and females are affected equally. Tumors do not express GLUT1, and approximately a third are diagnosed prenatally. The lesion is typically noted as an abdominal mass in a healthy neonate. Fifteen percent of children exhibit cutaneous infantile hemangiomas. Cardiac overload (25%) can occur, and intralesional thrombosis may result in transient anemia (25%) or thrombocytopenia (33%). MRI or CT shows a well-localized lesion with peripheral enhancement and central sparing because of thrombosis, necrosis, and/or intralesional bleeding. More than 90% volume reduction is achieved by 13 months of age. Tumor volume decreases 35% each month from 0 to 3 months of life, and then 12% per month between 3 and 6 months of life. Imaging shows a focal, heterogeneous, subcapsular lesion with peripheral hypervascularity. After involution, a small, calcified, subcapsular nodule may be present. Patients are not at risk for hypothyroidism, and treatment is rarely necessary. If high-output heart failure is present, patients can be treated with pharmacotherapy (corticosteroid, propranolol) or embolization while the tumor regresses.
- *Multifocal hepatic hemangiomas* are infantile hemangiomas that are most often accompanied by cutaneous lesions (77%). They are usually discovered during hepatic screening in an infant with hemangiomatosis (five or more cutaneous infantile hemangio-

mas). Liver tumors express GLUT1 and proliferate or involute similar to infantile hemangiomas involving the integument. Females (two thirds) are more commonly affected than males. Because all infantile hemangiomas develop postnatally, multifocal hepatic lesions cannot be diagnosed prenatally. On imaging, the hemangiomas are hyperintense and diffusely enhance. Normal hepatic parenchyma is present in between liver lesions. Although usually asymptomatic, the tumors can cause high-output cardiac failure, and 21% of infants develop hypothyroidism from type 3 iodothyronine deiodinase production. Patients should undergo thyroid-stimulating hormone screening to determine whether they require thyroid hormone replacement to prevent mental retardation and heart failure. Hypothyroidism resolves as the tumor involutes. Symptomatic lesions causing heart failure and/or hypothyroidism are managed with oral pharmacotherapy and/or embolization. Tumors are followed by serial ultrasound during the proliferative phase. After the infantile hemangiomas have regressed the previously involved liver parenchyma appears normal.

- *Diffuse hepatic hemangioma* is an infantile hemangioma that is often diagnosed during the neonatal period because of severe symptoms (massive hepatomegaly, respiratory compromise, abdominal compartment syndrome, and/or heart failure). A diffuse hepatic hemangioma does not exhibit normal hepatic parenchyma in between lesions (the liver is almost completely replaced by the tumor). A diffuse hepatic hemangioma may represent the more severe spectrum of enlarging multifocal lesions. Half of patients also have cutaneous hemangiomas, and females are more often affected (70%). Tumors immunostain for GLUT1 and cannot be visualized prenatally. All lesions cause hypothyroidism as a result of a large amount of tumor deiodinase production that inactivates thyroid hormone. Intravenous thyroid hormone replacement is given to prevent mental retardation and heart failure until the tumor regresses. Most patients are treated with pharmacotherapy (corticosteroid, propranolol) and/or embolization to prevent enlargement of the tumor and to stimulate accelerated regression.

Lumbosacral Location

- Infants with an isolated midline infantile hemangioma greater than 2.5 cm involving the lumbosacral skin have a 35% risk of having an underlying spinal anomaly. The association increases to 51% if another cutaneous marker of dysraphism is present (a sacral dimple, skin appendage, abnormal gluteal cleft, dermal sinus, lipoma, aplasia cutis, or dermal melanocytosis).
- The most common spinal anomalies are tethered cord (60%), lipoma (50%), and intraspinal hemangioma (45%); 40% of patients have a sinus tract.
- 85% of children with a spinal anomaly are asymptomatic.
- Ultrasound has a 50% false-negative rate for identifying an underlying spinal anomaly. Consequently, MRI is obtained between 3 and 6 months of age to rule out an occult spinal dysraphism.

PHACES Association

- This condition consists of a plaquelike infantile hemangioma in a "segmental" or trigeminal nerve distribution of the face with one or more of the following anomalies: *p*osterior fossa brain malformation, *h*emangioma, *a*rterial cerebrovascular anomalies, *c*oarctation of the aorta and cardiac defects, *e*ye/*e*ndocrine abnormalities, *s*ternal clefting/*s*upraumbilical raphe.
- The hemangioma often exhibits minimal postnatal growth.
- Affects 2.3% of children with infantile hemangioma; 90% are female.
- Cerebrovascular anomalies are the most common associated finding (72%).
- One third of children have more than one extracutaneous feature.
- 8% have a stroke in infancy, and 42% have a structural brain anomaly.

- MRI is used to evaluate the cerebrovasculature. If an anomaly is present, neurologic consultation is obtained, and aspirin is considered to reduce the risk of stroke.
- Ophthalmologic, endocrine, and cardiac evaluation are performed to rule out associated anomalies.

LUMBAR Association

- LUMBAR association describes a *l*ower body infantile hemangioma, *u*rogenital anomalies or *u*lceration, *m*yelopathy, *b*ony deformities, *a*norectal malformations or *a*rterial anomalies, and *r*enal anomalies.
- Females (63%) are typically affected.
- The infantile hemangioma is extensive, superficial, plaquelike, and located in a "segmental" or regional distribution. Unlike a typical infantile hemangioma, the lesion has minimal postnatal growth and a higher risk of ulceration (70%). The infantile hemangioma expresses GLUT1.
- The tumor affects the sacral area (83%), lumbar region (75%), perineum/genitals (67%), and/or the lower extremity (42%). Two thirds of lesions involve more than one region, and many affect all four areas.
- Associated anomalies include myelopathy (83%), cutaneous (45%), anorectal (29%), renal (25%), urogenital (21%), arterial (8%), and bone (8%).
- 30% of patients have only one associated anomaly.
- Patients with a myelopathy (usually a tethered cord and lipomyelocele/lipomyelomeningocele) typically have an infantile hemangioma in the lumbar area.
- The most frequent type of anorectal malformation is an imperforate anus, and all patients have an infantile hemangioma involving the sacral region.
- The typical renal abnormality is a solitary kidney, and patients have an infantile hemangioma located in the sacral area.

- All patients with urogenital anomalies, such as bladder extrophy, ureter reflux, vaginal atresia, undescended testis, or hypospadias, have an infantile hemangioma located in the sacral region.
- Bony deformities of the lower extremity or pelvis are associated with an infantile hemangioma of the limb.
- Diffuse, reticular/"segmental" infantile hemangiomas involving the lower extremity are associated with atrophy of the limb as well as underlying arterial anomalies, such as a hypoplastic ilio-femoral artery, aberrant arterial course or origin, or persistence of embryonic anastomoses.
- Management of an infant suspected of having LUMBAR association includes the following:
  - If the patient is less than 3 months of age, a screening ultrasound is performed of the spine, abdomen, and pelvis to search for large anomalies and spinal dysraphism.
  - When the infant is more than 3 months of age, an MRI of the spine, abdomen, and pelvis is conducted, because the false-negative rate of screening ultrasound is high, and the risk of sedation for the MRI is lower after 3 months of age.
  - If the lower limb is involved, an MRI/MRA is ordered when the infant is more than 3 months of age to rule out arterial limb anomalies.

MANAGEMENT

Observation

- Most children with infantile hemangioma are observed, because 90% of lesions are small, localized, and do not involve important areas.
- Infants are followed monthly during the proliferative phase if the tumor has the potential to become problematic (for example, may cause obstruction or destruction of important structures).
- During involution, patients are followed annually if intervention may be necessary in childhood to improve a deformity.

Wound Care

- 16% of infantile hemangiomas will ulcerate at a median age of 4 months. Lip, neck, and anogenital tumors are most likely to ulcerate.
- To reduce the risk of ulceration, lesions are covered with hydrated petroleum to minimize desiccation and protect against shearing of the skin.
- Infantile hemangiomas in the anogenital area may be further protected with a petroleum gauze barrier to minimize friction from the diaper.
- If an ulceration develops, the wound is washed with soap and water at least twice daily. Small, superficial areas are managed with topical antibiotic ointment and occasionally with a petroleum gauze barrier. Large, deep wounds require damp-to-dry dressing changes. If bleeding occurs, it is minor and can be controlled with pressure.
- To minimize discomfort, a small amount of topical lidocaine may be applied, no more than four times daily to avoid toxicity. A *e*utectic *m*ixture of *l*ocal *a*nesthetics (EMLA) contains prilocaine and should not be used in infants less than 3 months of age, because it can cause methemoglobinemia.
- Almost all ulcerations will heal with local wound care and the elimination of extrinsic factors that may have contributed to the ulceration, such as desiccation or trauma.
- If an ulceration fails to heal with conservative measures, intralesional or oral pharmacotherapy may be necessary to provide a more favorable intrinsic environment for wound healing.

Topical Corticosteroid

- A topical corticosteroid has minimal efficacy, especially when the infantile hemangioma involves the deep dermis and subcutis.
- Ultrapotent agents such as clobetasol propionate 0.05% may be effective for small, superficial lesions, particularly in the peri-

orbital area. Although lightening of the skin may occur, if an underlying mass is present, it will not be affected. Adverse effects include hypopigmentation and skin atrophy.

Topical Timolol

- Topical timolol may be effective for small, superficial infantile hemangiomas in unfavorable locations, such as the periorbital area, lip, or nose. The drug does not penetrate through the dermis, and thus deep tumors are not affected.
- Timolol 0.5% gel-forming solution (5 mg/ml) applied twice daily may prevent proliferation and cause accelerated regression. Some authors apply the medication more than twice daily (the half-life is 4 hours) and/or use an occlusive dressing in an attempt to increase its efficacy.
- Asthma, apnea, and bradycardia have occurred following ophthalmologic use of timolol as a result of systemic absorption of the drug. Although these complications have not been reported when used for infantile hemangioma, patients should be screened for pulmonary or cardiac disease before topical timolol is used.
- Dermatologic side effects include alopecia, rash, and urticaria.
- Timolol is 10 times more potent than propranolol, and systemic absorption occurs when it is applied topically. It should not be used more than twice daily in areas where absorption is greater (including the eyelids, mucosa, or an ulcerated tumor).
- It has been estimated that each drop of topical timolol (0.05 ml) has at least a systemic bioavailability of 50% and is minimally equivalent to 2 mg of oral propranolol. Consequently, the number of drops applied to the hemangioma should be precise (1 or 2 drops).

Intralesional Corticosteroid

- An intralesional corticosteroid is indicated for small, well-localized infantile hemangiomas that obstruct the visual axis or nasal airway, are at risk for damaging aesthetically sensitive structures, such as the eyelid, lip, or nose, or may cause a significant deformity in an unfavorable location, such as the face (Fig. 3-3).
- Triamcinolone (40 mg/ml) stabilizes growth in 95% of infantile hemangiomas, and 75% will decrease in size.
- The injection is delivered using a 1 ml syringe and 30-gauge needle. The dose should not exceed 3 mg/kg for each injection and lasts 4 to 6 weeks.
- Patients are evaluated 4 to 6 weeks after the injection. If the child is less than 6 months of age and/or the infantile hemangioma has exhibited rebound growth since the last injection, another injection is considered.
- Risks include subcutaneous fat atrophy (approximately 1%) or ulceration (less than 3%). Adrenal suppression may occur after large-volume injections, although adverse sequelae have not been described. Cases of blindness have been reported after injection of an upper eyelid infantile hemangioma, possibly

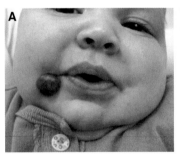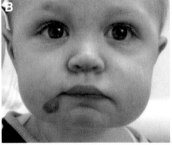

Fig. 3-3 Management of problematic infantile hemangioma with corticosteroid injection. **A,** A 2½-month-old girl with a well-localized, rapidly enlarging tumor in an unfavorable location. The lesion was injected with corticosteroid. **B,** The infantile hemangioma has undergone accelerated involution at 11 months of age.

as a result of embolic occlusion of the retinal artery. However, no visual problems have been recorded following injection of triamcinolone.

- If a localized lesion fails to respond to intralesional corticosteroid treatment, systemic pharmacotherapy is considered.

Systemic Pharmacotherapy

- Systemic pharmacotherapy is indicated for problematic infantile hemangiomas that cannot be managed with an intralesional corticosteroid (a lesion that is diffuse, greater than 3 cm in diameter, or has failed corticosteroid injection) (Fig. 3-4).
- There are two primary drug options: prednisolone (a corticosteroid) and propranolol (a beta-blocker).
    - Prednisolone has been a first-line systemic pharmacotherapy for problematic infantile hemangioma since 1967. A dose of 3 mg/kg is given once in the morning for 1 month. The dose is then tapered by 0.5 ml every 2 to 4 weeks until it is discontinued between 10 and 12 months of age. Nearly 100% of infantile hemangiomas will stop growing, and 88% will become

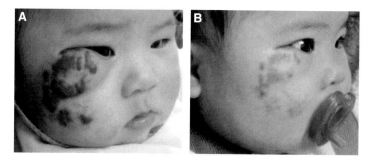

Fig. 3-4   Management of problematic hemangioma with systemic pharmacotherapy. **A,** A 4-month-old girl with a large, rapidly growing tumor causing a significant deformity and affecting vision. The child was treated with prednisolone. **B,** Accelerated involution of the infantile hemangioma at 12 months of age.

smaller. Twenty percent develop a cushingoid appearance that resolves when the drug is weaned, and 12% of infants have a temporary decrease in their gain in height, but return to their pretreatment growth curve by 24 months of age. Gastric and antibiotic prophylaxis is not required. Complicated monitoring is unnecessary. The dose is rapidly tapered as the infant gains weight. Patients are followed monthly in the office, and the dose is lowered further. If rebound growth of the tumor occurs, the dose is increased.

– Propranolol (1 to 3 mg/kg/day) has been popularized since 2008. A total of 2 mg/kg/day is divided into three daily doses and then tapered until it is discontinued between 10 and 12 months of age. The drug is started at 1 mg/kg/day and then slowly increased to 2 mg/kg/day. Approximately 90% of tumors stop growing or regress. Risks (less than 3%) include bronchospasm, bradycardia, hypotension, hypoglycemia, seizures, and hyperkalemia. Preterm infants and children less than 3 months of age are more likely to have an adverse event (particularly hypoglycemia, because their glucose utilization is higher during fasting and they have lower glycogen reserves). Patients typically have a cardiology consultation (75%) and undergo an electrocardiogram (81%), echocardiogram (38%), glucose/electrolyte measurements, and frequent blood pressure, heart rate, and respiratory examinations. Children with airway disease, those born prematurely, or infants less than 3 months of age often undergo inpatient initiation of drug treatment. Potential contraindications include asthma or reactive airway disease, glucose abnormalities, congenital heart disease, hypotension, bradycardia, or cerebrovascular malformations (PHACES association). A 2013 consensus statement recommended that (1) an electrocardiogram should be obtained before treatment (especially if the child has a low heart rate, a family history of cardiac disease, or abnormal findings on cardiac examination), (2) routine echocardiography is unnecessary, (3) doses should be divided three times daily to reduce the risk of adverse events, (4) inpatient initiation of treatment is appropriate for infants 8 weeks of age or younger or with comorbidities, (5) heart rate and blood pressure should be measured (baseline, 1 hour, 2 hours) after the initial dose, a dose escalation of more than 0.5 mg/kg/day, and following the final target dose of 2 mg/kg/day, (6) routine glucose screening is not indicated; infants should be fed immediately after receiving propranolol, and fasting longer than 5 hours is avoided, and (7) propranolol should be discontinued if the infant is ill, because reduced oral intake can increase the risk of hypoglycemia. The maximum effect of propranolol on the cardiovasculature is 2 hours following administration. The physiologic response is greatest after the first dose; thus repeat heart rate and blood pressure monitoring in a healthy patient is unnecessary. Heart rate measurement is most predictive of the cardiac effect of propranolol, because blood pressure monitoring in neonates and infants is difficult (bradycardia in an infant 1 to 12 months of age is less than 80 beats/minute).

- Prednisolone and propranolol should not be administered at the same time, because the risk of hypoglycemia is increased. Corticosteroid administration may reduce the adrenal cortisol response to propranolol-induced hypoglycemia.
- Interferon is no longer recommended in children less than 12 months of age, because it can cause neurologic problems, particularly spastic diplegia.
- Vincristine may be considered in the unlikely event that a child has failed or has a contraindication to prednisolone and propranolol.

Embolic Therapy

- Embolization is rarely indicated for the initial control of heart failure (usually hepatic hemangiomas) while the therapeutic effects of systemic pharmacotherapy are pending.

Laser Therapy

- Pulsed-dye laser treatment during the proliferating phase is contraindicated. The laser only reaches the superficial portion of the tumor—it can penetrate up to 1.2 mm into the dermis—and although lightening may result, the mass is not affected. Ulceration and hypopigmentation can occur, because the ischemic dermis cannot tolerate the thermal injury delivered by the laser.
- Pulsed-dye laser effectively eliminates residual telangiectasias once the infantile hemangioma has completed involution.
- Carbon dioxide laser may be useful for the treatment of an infantile hemangioma involving the airway.

Operative Treatment

Proliferative Phase

- Operative intervention is rarely indicated during infancy, because problematic lesions can be successfully managed with intralesional or systemic pharmacotherapy.
- The tumor is highly vascular during this period, and the patient is at risk for blood loss, iatrogenic injury, and an inferior aesthetic outcome, compared with resection after the tumor has regressed.
- Anesthetic morbidity is three to eight times greater in infants, compared with children older than 1 year of age.
- Factors that lower the threshold for excision include the following:
  - Failure or contraindication to pharmacotherapy
  - A well-localized lesion in an anatomically safe area
  - Complicated reconstruction not required
  - Resection will be necessary in the future and the appearance of the area would be similar

Involuted Phase

- Operative intervention after 3 years of age is much safer than excision during the proliferative phase, because the lesion is smaller and less vascular (Fig. 3-5).
- 50% of infantile hemangiomas leave a permanent deformity once they have finished involuting: postulceration scarring, alopecia, anetoderma, expanded skin, fibrofatty residuum, and destroyed structures, such as the nose, ear, or lip.
- Because the lesion has been allowed to shrink maximally, the extent of the excision and reconstruction is reduced, and thus the aesthetic outcome is superior.

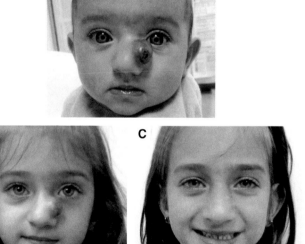

Fig. 3-5   Timing of operative intervention for infantile hemangioma. **A,** A 6-month-old girl with a large tumor of the nose. **B,** At 3 years of age, the hemangioma has regressed, leaving residual fibrofatty tissue and excess skin. Resection was performed at this time, rather than during infancy, to allow the lesion to become smaller and less vascular. **C,** One year after circular excision and purse-string closure of the involuted hemangioma.

- It is preferable to intervene surgically between 3 and 4 years of age. During this period the infantile hemangioma will no longer improve significantly, and the procedure is performed before the child's long-term memory and self-esteem begin to form at about 4 years of age. Some parents may elect to wait until the child is older and able to make the decision to proceed with operative intervention, especially if the deformity is minor.

Operative Principles and Techniques

- Before excision the area should be infiltrated with local anesthetic containing epinephrine to minimize blood loss and iatrogenic injury.
- Because the tumor acts as a tissue expander, there is usually adequate skin to allow primary, linear closure of the wound (Fig. 3-6).
- Circular lesions, particularly on the face, are best treated by a two-stage circular excision and purse-string closure. During the first procedure the infantile hemangioma is removed and the

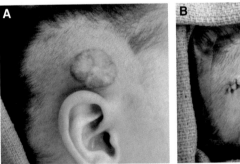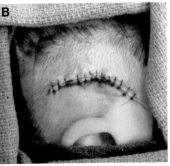

Fig. 3-6 Operative management of infantile hemangioma using lenticular excision. **A,** A 4-year-old girl with an involuted infantile hemangioma of the scalp that has left residual fibrofatty tissue and excess skin. **B,** Following resection of the tumor using a lenticular incision. Note that the scar is approximately twice the length of the diameter of the infantile hemangioma.

wound is closed with a purse-string suture (Fig. 3-7). The resulting circular scar can be removed 6 to 12 months later and closed linearly. This method minimizes the length of the scar to approximately the same diameter as the originally excised infantile hemangioma. If a circular lesion is removed using a lenticular excision, the resulting linear scar is three times the diameter of the lesion. After the first stage, 50% of families will not elect to

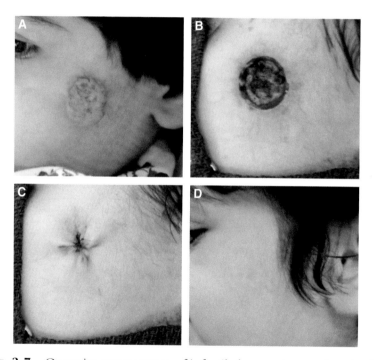

Fig. 3-7   Operative management of infantile hemangioma using circular excision and purse-string closure. **A,** A 2½-year-old girl with an involuted infantile hemangioma of the cheek with fibrofatty residuum and excess skin. Because the tumor was located in an unfavorable location, it was removed using a circular excision and purse-string closure to limit the length of the scar. **B,** Following resection of the tumor. **C,** Purse-string closure of the wound. **D,** Favorable scar 1 year postoperatively.

proceed to the second stage to convert the circular scar into a line, because the circular scar can be difficult to appreciate (it can resemble an acne or chicken-pox scar). The disadvantages of circular excision and purse-string closure are that:

— Temporary bunching of the skin occurs (this resolves after several weeks).
— A second stage may be required.

• In the scalp, lenticular excision and linear closure are preferred to circular excision and purse-string closure because:

— The length of a linear scar in the scalp is not critical because it is covered by hair.
— The procedure is one stage.
— The scalp lacks the skin redundancy necessary for purse-string closure.
— A circular scar in the scalp may cause a visible area of alopecia.

Selected References

Arnold R, Chaudry G. Diagnostic imaging of vascular anomalies. Clin Plast Surg 38:21-29, 2011.

Bennett ML, Fleischer AB, Chamlin SL, Frieden IJ. Oral corticosteroid use is effective for cutaneous hemangiomas. Arch Dermatol 137:1208-1213, 2001.

Chang LC, Haggstrom AN, Drolet BA, Baselga E, Chamlin SL, Garzon MC, Horii KA, Lucky AW, Mancini AJ, Metry DW, Nopper AJ, Frieden IJ. Growth characteristics of infantile hemangiomas: implications for management. Pediatrics 122:360-367, 2008.

Couto RA, Maclellan RA, Zurakowski D, Greene AK. Infantile hemangioma: clinical assessment of the involuting phase and implications for management. Plast Reconstr Surg 130:619-624, 2012.

Drolet BA, Chamlin SL, Garzon MC, Adams D, Baselga E, Haggstrom AN, Holland KE, Horii KA, Juern A, Lucky AW, Mancini AJ, McCuaig C, Metry DW, Morel KD, Newell BD, Nopper AJ, Powell J, Frieden IJ. Prospective study of spinal anomalies in children with infantile hemangiomas of the lumbosacral skin. J Pediatr 157:789-794, 2010.

Drolet BA, Frommelt PC, Chamlin SL, Haggstrom A, Bauman NM, Chiu YE, Chun RH, Garzon MC, Holland KE, Liberman L, Maclellan-Tobert S, Mancini AJ, Metry D, Puttgen KB, Seefeldt M, Sidbury R, Ward KM, Blei F, Baselga E, Cassidy L, Darrow DH, Joachim S, Kwon EK, Martin K, Perkins J, Siegel DH, Boucek RJ, Frieden IJ. Initiation and use of propranolol for infantile hemangioma: report of a consensus conference. Pediatrics 131:128-140, 2013.

Greene AK. Management of hemangiomas and other vascular tumors. Clin Plast Surg 38:45-63, 2011.

Greene AK, Couto RA. Oral prednisolone for infantile hemangioma: efficacy and safety using a standardized treatment protocol. Plast Reconstr Surg 128:743-752, 2011.

Gupta A, Kozakewich H. Histopathology of vascular anomalies. Clin Plast Surg 38:31-44, 2011.

Horii KA, Drolet BA, Frieden IJ, Baselga E, Chamlin SL, Haggstrom AN, Holland KE, Mancini AJ, McCuaig CC, Metry DW, Morel KD, Newell BD, Nopper AJ, Powell J, Garzon MC. Prospective study of the frequency of hepatic hemangiomas in infants with multiple cutaneous infantile hemangiomas. Pediatr Dermatol 28:245-253, 2011.

Huang SA, Tu HM, Harney JW, Venihaki M, Butte AJ, Kozakewich HP, Fishman SJ, Larsen PR. Severe hypothyroidism caused by type 3 iodothyronine deiodinase in infantile hemangiomas. N Engl J Med 343:185-189, 2000.

Iacobas I, Burrows PE, Frieden IJ, Liang MG, Mulliken JB, Mancini AJ, Kramer D, Paller AS, Silverman R, Wagner AM, Metry DW. LUMBAR: association between cutaneous infantile hemangiomas of the lower body and regional congenital anomalies. J Pediatr 157:795-801, 2010.

Kulungowski AM, Alomari AI, Chawla A, Christison-Lagay ER, Fishman SJ. Lessons from a liver hemangioma registry: subtype classification. J Pediatr Surg 47:165-170, 2012.

Léauté-Labrèze C, Dumas de la Roque E, Hubiche T, Boralevi F, Thambo JB, Taïeb A. Propranolol for severe hemangiomas of infancy. N Engl J Med 358:2649-2651, 2008.

McMahon P, Oza V, Frieden IJ. Topical timolol for infantile hemangiomas: putting a note of caution in "cautiously optimistic." Pediatr Dermatol 29:127-130, 2012.

Metry DW, Garzon MC, Drolet BA, Frommelt P, Haggstrom A, Hall J, Hess CP, Heyer GL, Siegel D, Baselga E, Katowitz W, Levy ML, Mancini A, Maronn ML, Phung T, Pope E, Sun G, Frieden IJ. PHACE syndrome: current knowledge, future directions. Pediatr Dermatol 26:381-398, 2009.

North PE, Waner M, Mizeracki A, Mihm MC Jr. GLUT1: a newly discovered immunohistochemical marker for juvenile hemangiomas. Hum Pathol 31:11-22, 2000.

Sans V, Dumas de la Roque E, Berge J, Grenier N, Boralevi F, Mazereeuw-Hautier J, Lipsker D, Dupuis E, Ezzedine K, Vergnes P, Taïeb A, Léauté-Labrèze C. Propranolol for severe infantile hemangiomas: follow-up report. Pediatrics 124:423-431, 2009.

CHAPTER 4

Congenital Hemangioma

TUMORS	MALFORMATIONS		
	Slow-Flow	**Fast-Flow**	**Overgrowth Syndromes**
Infantile Hemangioma	*Capillary Malformation*	*Arteriovenous Malformation*	CLOVES Klippel-Trenaunay Maffucci Parkes Weber Proteus Sturge-Weber
Congenital Hemangioma Rapidly involuting Noninvoluting	*Lymphatic Malformation*		
Kaposiform Hemangioendothelioma	*Venous Malformation*		
Pyogenic Granuloma			
Rare Vascular Tumors			

CLINICAL FEATURES

- A congenital hemangioma (CH) forms in utero and is fully grown at birth. It does not undergo postnatal enlargement.
- There are two types: rapidly involuting congenital hemangioma (RICH) and noninvoluting congenital hemangioma (NICH).
  - A RICH involutes immediately after birth: 50% complete regression by 7 months of age, and the remainder fully involute by 14 months. A RICH affects the head and neck (42%), limbs (52%), or trunk (6%). Unlike infantile hemangioma, which commonly leaves excess fibrofatty tissue following involution, a RICH may result in atrophic skin and deficient subcutaneous adipose tissue after it has regressed (Fig. 4-1).
  - A NICH does not undergo postnatal regression and remains unchanged. It involves the head and neck (43%), limbs (38%), or trunk (19%) (Fig. 4-2).

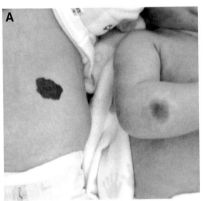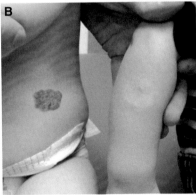

Fig. 4-1 Comparison of infantile hemangioma and congenital hemangioma. **A,** Twins at 6 weeks of age. Note the red, superficial infantile hemangioma on the abdomen of one child, and the purple congenital hemangioma (with a surrounding pale halo) on the extremity of the sibling. **B,** At 12 months of age, the infantile hemangioma is beginning involution, while the congenital hemangioma (RICH) has fully regressed.

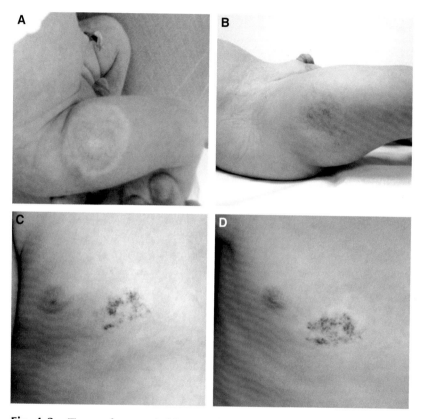

Fig. 4-2 Types of congenital hemangiomas. **A,** A 2-week-old infant with a rapidly involuting congenital hemangioma (RICH) of the lower extremity. **B,** Complete regression of the tumor at 12 months of age. Note subcutaneous fat atrophy, in contrast to an infantile hemangioma, which commonly leaves excess adipose tissue following involution. **C,** A 12-month-old girl with a noninvoluting congenital hemangioma (NICH) that was present at birth. **D,** The tumor has not regressed and persists at 4 years of age.

DIAGNOSIS

History and Physical Examination

- Because congenital hemangiomas develop during fetal life, occasionally they may be identified during prenatal ultrasonography.
- 95% of congenital hemangiomas can be diagnosed by history and physical examination.
- The primary differential diagnosis includes other fast-flow vascular anomalies: infantile hemangioma, kaposiform hemangioendothelioma, or arteriovenous malformation.
- Unlike infantile hemangioma, the lesion is fully grown at birth and has a more violaceous appearance, with coarse telangiectasias and a peripheral pale halo.
- Unlike infantile hemangioma, congenital hemangiomas:
  - More commonly affect the extremities
  - Have an equal sex distribution
  - Are always solitary
  - Are typically large (average diameter 5 cm)
- The type of congenital hemangioma (RICH or NICH) often cannot be determined at birth, although a RICH is more likely to have soft tissue overgrowth and a NICH is typically flat.
- RICH and NICH are differentiated by their clinical behavior over the first months of life. If the lesion becomes smaller after birth, it is a RICH; if it remains unchanged during infancy, the tumor is a NICH.
- Handheld Doppler examination will show fast-flow and can differentiate congenital hemangiomas from slow-flow vascular malformations (capillary, lymphatic, or venous).

Imaging

- Imaging is rarely indicated for diagnosis.
- It is difficult to differentiate a congenital hemangioma from an infantile hemangioma radiographically.

- On ultrasound, congenital hemangiomas have less-defined borders and are more likely to contain larger vessels, thrombi, calcifications, and shunting compared with infantile hemangiomas.
- The MRI appearance of a congenital hemangioma and an infantile hemangioma is very similar.

Histopathology

- Biopsy is rarely required for diagnosis of a congenital hemangioma.
- A RICH shows lobules of capillaries containing thickened, irregular fibromuscular walls surrounded by abundant fibrous stroma. The basement membranes are thin, and endothelial cells are moderately plump. In the center of the lesion few lobules and large draining vessels (representative of involution) are present. Hematopoiesis, arteriovenous shunting, aneurysms, hemosiderin, and thrombi are occasionally noted.
- A NICH contains large lobules of thin-walled capillaries, with larger channels than are present in a RICH. Endothelial cells have minimal cytoplasm that contains eosinophilic globules. Nuclei protrude into the vessel lumen. Interlobular fibrous tissue is prominent and contains large arteries and veins with fistulas.
- RICH and NICH do not stain for GLUT1 and thus can be differentiated from infantile hemangioma immunohistochemically.

MANAGEMENT

Rapidly Involuting Congenital Hemangioma

- A RICH almost never requires intervention in infancy, because it rapidly involutes. Lesions are observed.
- Rarely, large tumors can cause congestive heart failure, which is managed by systemic corticosteroid or embolization as the lesion involutes.

- Reconstruction of damaged skin or atrophic subcutaneous tissue can begin before 4 years of age, when memory and self-esteem begin to form. Alternatively, some families may elect to wait until the child wishes to have the area improved later in childhood or adolescence.
  - Reconstruction of atrophic subcutaneous tissue with autologous dermis, fat grafts, or acellular dermis may be indicated (Fig. 4-3). Residual telangiectasias can be lightened with a pulsed-dye laser.

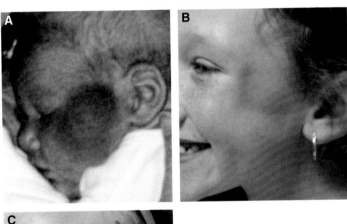

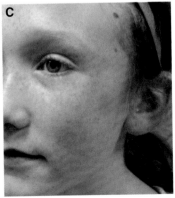

Fig. 4-3 Operative management of a RICH. **A,** Newborn girl with a RICH involving the left side of the face. **B,** At 8 years of age, the girl was unhappy with residual subcutaneous atrophy of her cheek. **C,** Eighteen months after fat grafting to the area.

Noninvoluting Congenital Hemangioma

- A NICH is rarely problematic in infancy and is observed. A symptomatic lesion is managed by embolization or resection.
- A NICH does not regress, and thus it can cause psychosocial morbidity by leaving a visible deformity.
- Resection may be indicated to improve the appearance of the affected area (Fig. 4-4). If the lesion is large, serial excision may be necessary.
- Pulsed-dye laser and/or sclerotherapy can improve the appearance of a NICH by eliminating telangiectasias.
- Parents may elect to have a visible lesion excised before the patient is 4 years of age, prior to the onset of memory and self-esteem. Alternatively, they may wait until the child is old enough to make his or her own decision to remove the lesion.

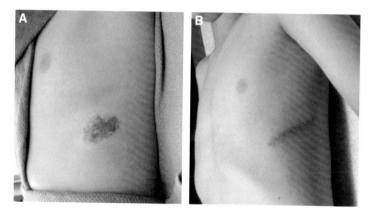

Fig. 4-4   Operative management of a NICH. **A,** This 8-year-old boy was unhappy with the appearance of a NICH on his trunk. **B,** Four weeks after resection.

Selected References

Arnold R, Chaudry G. Diagnostic imaging of vascular anomalies. Clin Plast Surg 38:21-29, 2011.

Berenguer B, Mulliken JB, Enjolras O, Boon LM, Wassef M, Josset P, Burrows PE, Perez-Atayde AR, Kozakewich HP. Rapidly involuting congenital hemangioma: clinical and histopathologic features. Pediatr Dev Pathol 6:495-510, 2003.

Boon LM, Enjolras O, Mulliken JB. Congenital hemangioma: evidence of accelerated involution. J Pediatr 128:329-335, 1996.

Enjolras O, Mulliken JB, Boon LM, Wassef M, Kozakewich HP, Burrows PE. Noninvoluting congenital hemangioma: a rare cutaneous vascular anomaly. Plast Reconstr Surg 107:1647-1654, 2001.

Greene AK. Management of hemangiomas and other vascular tumors. Clin Plast Surg 38:45-63, 2011.

Gupta A, Kozakewich H. Histopathology of vascular anomalies. Clin Plast Surg 38:31-44, 2011.

Kaposiform Hemangioendothelioma

TUMORS	MALFORMATIONS		
	Slow-Flow	Fast-Flow	Overgrowth Syndromes
Infantile Hemangioma	*Capillary Malformation*	*Arteriovenous Malformation*	CLOVES Klippel-Trenaunay Maffucci Parkes Weber Proteus Sturge-Weber
Congenital Hemangioma	*Lymphatic Malformation*		
Kaposiform Hemangioendothelioma	*Venous Malformation*		
Pyogenic Granuloma			
Rare Vascular Tumors			

CLINICAL FEATURES

- Kaposiform hemangioendothelioma (KHE) is a rare vascular neoplasm that is locally aggressive but does not metastasize (Fig. 5-1).
- Prevalence is approximately 1/100,000 children.
- 60% of these neoplasms are noted in the neonatal period, and 93% present during infancy. Patients also may be diagnosed in childhood. Adult onset can occur as well (the mean age is 42.9 years, and 80% of those affected are male).
- Lesions appear reddish–purple and are solitary, flat, and painful.
- Often greater than 5 cm and involves multiple tissue planes.
- Equal sex distribution, and affects the head and neck (40%), trunk (30%), or extremity (30%).
- Slowly enlarges in early childhood and then partially regresses after 2 years of age.
- Usually persists long-term, causing chronic pain, stiffness, and contractures.
- 71% of affected patients have life-threatening Kasabach-Merritt phenomenon (thrombocytopenia with a platelet count below $25,000/mm^3$, petechiae, and bleeding).
- Those with retroperitoneal, intrathoracic, or muscle involvement have an 85% or higher risk of Kasabach-Merritt phenomenon. Patients with lesions smaller than 8 cm or with onset after infancy are less likely to develop Kasabach-Merritt phenomenon.
- Kaposiform hemangioendothelioma has overlapping clinical and histopathologic features with another tumor, tufted angioma. Tufted angioma has an anatomic distribution similar to that of kaposiform hemangioendothelioma, but it is more erythematous and plaquelike.

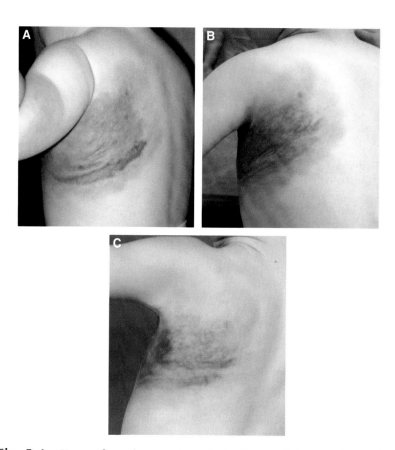

Fig. 5-1   Kaposiform hemangioendothelioma of the trunk causing Kasabach-Merritt phenomenon. **A,** At 11 months of age. **B,** At 3 years of age, the tumor has regressed following treatment with vincristine. **C,** At 5 years, the lesion continues to improve naturally.

DIAGNOSIS

History and Physical Examination

- 90% are diagnosed by history and physical examination.
- Kaposiform hemangioendothelioma is typically present at birth and does not exhibit rapid postnatal growth.
- Lesions are reddish-purple, painful, superficial, and involve wide areas and multiple tissue planes.
- Kasabach-Merritt phenomenon is pathognomonic for kaposiform hemangioendothelioma.

Imaging

- Patients undergo MRI for diagnostic confirmation and to evaluate the extent of the tumor.
- MRI shows poorly defined margins, small vessels, and invasion of adjacent tissues.
- Kaposiform hemangioendothelioma is hypointense/isointense on T1 sequences and hyperintense on T2 images. Lesions enhance heterogeneously with contrast.
- Lymphatic involvement causes subcutaneous fat stranding, which is a unique feature that can differentiate kaposiform hemangioendothelioma from other fast-flow lesions.
- Prominent vessels and hemosiderin can cause signal voids.

Histopathology

- Kaposiform hemangioendothelioma is an infiltrative lesion with lobules containing round or spindled endothelial cells and pericytes. The tumor can have a glomeruloid appearance. The stroma contains edematous fluid, myxoid change, and fibrosis. Thrombi are present within capillaries, and cells contain hemosiderin. Foci of larger channels can be present, and thin-walled vessels usually surround the lobules. Hemosiderin-filled slitlike vascular spaces are present, with red blood cell fragments and dilated lymphatics.

- Mitoses and nuclear atypia are uncommon. Ki-67 (a proliferation marker) shows a low proliferative index.
- Kaposiform hemangioendothelioma can have dilated lymphatic channels, and the spindled cells immunostain for the lymphatic markers D240 and PROX1.

MANAGEMENT

Nonoperative Treatment

- Most kaposiform hemangioendotheliomas are symptomatic (pain, stiffness, deformity, Kasabach-Merritt phenomenon) and are treated with systemic pharmacotherapy until they "burn out" after 2 years of age.
- Because kaposiform hemangioendothelioma is typically diffuse and involves multiple tissue planes, resection is rarely possible.
- First-line treatment is vincristine (0.05 to 0.065 mg/kg intravenously weekly for 6 months) which has a greater than 90% response rate. Even without Kasabach-Merritt phenomenon, children with large tumors are treated with vincristine to minimize fibrosis and the risk of long-term pain, stiffness, and contractures.
- Second-line drugs include interferon (approximately 50% response rate) or a corticosteroid (approximately 10% response rate).
- Recently, sirolimus has shown favorable results for patients with kaposiform hemangioendothelioma and tufted angioma. The oral dose is 0.8 mg/m^2, divided into two daily doses. The goal trough level is 10 to 15 ng/ml.
- Platelet transfusion should be avoided in patients with Kasabach-Merritt phenomenon unless there is active bleeding or a surgical procedure is planned. Thrombocytopenia does not improve after transfusion: platelets are trapped in the lesion, and the size of the tumor increases as a result of swelling.
- Heparin is not given because it can stimulate growth of kaposiform hemangioendothelioma, aggravate platelet trapping, and worsen bleeding.

- By 2 years of age, the tumor often undergoes partial involution, and the platelet count normalizes in patients with Kasabach-Merritt phenomenon.

Operative Treatment

- Most patients have diffuse tumors involving multiple tissue planes and important structures that are difficult to resect. The majority of kaposiform hemangioendotheliomas are best managed with chemotherapy until they "burn out" in early childhood.
- Resection is not required for asymptomatic lesions without functional problems, because kaposiform hemangioendothelioma is benign.
- Small or localized tumors may be excised, particularly if there is a contraindication to or failure of pharmacotherapy. Wide margins are not necessary, because kaposiform hemangioendothelioma is not malignant.
- Reconstruction for secondary deformities caused by the tumor, such as contractures, may be necessary in childhood.

Selected References

Arnold R, Chaudry G. Diagnostic imaging of vascular anomalies. Clin Plast Surg 38:21-29, 2011.

Croteau SE, Liang MG, Kozakewich HP, Alomari AI, Fishman SJ, Mulliken JB, Trenor CC III. Kaposiform hemangioendothelioma: atypical features and risks of Kasabach-Merritt phenomenon in 107 referrals. J Pediatr (in press).

Greene AK. Management of hemangiomas and other vascular tumors. Clin Plast Surg 38:45-63, 2011.

Gupta A, Kozakewich H. Histopathology of vascular anomalies. Clin Plast Surg 38:31-44, 2011.

Haisley-Royster C, Enjolras O, Frieden IJ, Garzon M, Lee M, Oranje A, de Laat PC, Madern GC, Gonzalez F, Frangoul H, Le Moine P, Prose NS, Adams DM. Kasabach-Merritt phenomenon: a retrospective study of treatment with vincristine. J Pediatr Hematol Oncol 24:459-462, 2002.

Lyons LL, North PE, Mac-Moune Lai F, Stoler MH, Folpe AL, Weiss SW. Kaposiform hemangioendothelioma: a study of 33 cases emphasizing its pathologic, immunophenotypic, and biologic uniqueness from juvenile hemangioma. Am J Surg Pathol 28:559-568, 2004.

Mulliken JB, Anupindi S, Ezekowitz RA, Mihm MC Jr. Case 13-2004: a newborn girl with a large cutaneous lesion, thrombocytopenia, and anemia. N Engl J Med 350:1764-1775, 2004.

Sarkar M, Mulliken JB, Kozakewich HP, Robertson RL, Burrows PE. Thrombocytopenic coagulopathy (Kasabach-Merritt phenomenon) is associated with kaposiform hemangioendothelioma and not with common infantile hemangioma. Plast Reconstr Surg 100:1377-1386, 1997.

Zukerberg LR, Nikoloff BJ, Weiss SW. Kaposiform hemangioendothelioma of infancy and childhood: an aggressive neoplasm associated with Kasabach-Merritt syndrome and lymphangiomatosis. Am J Surg Pathol 17:321-328, 1993.

CHAPTER 6

Pyogenic Granuloma

TUMORS	MALFORMATIONS		
	Slow-Flow	Fast-Flow	Overgrowth Syndromes
Infantile Hemangioma	*Capillary Malformation*	*Arteriovenous Malformation*	CLOVES Klippel-Trenaunay Maffucci Parkes Weber Proteus Sturge-Weber
Congenital Hemangioma	*Lymphatic Malformation*		
Kaposiform Hemangioendothelioma	*Venous Malformation*		
Pyogenic Granuloma			
Rare Vascular Tumors			

CLINICAL FEATURES

- Pyogenic granuloma (PG) has also been called *lobular capillary hemangioma.*
- It is common and acquired, although congenital and multifocal lesions have been described.
- Pyogenic granuloma is a solitary red papule that grows rapidly and typically forms a stalk (Fig. 6-1).
- The average diameter is 6.5 mm (range 2 to 20 mm), and 75% are less than 1 cm.
- Bleeding is common (64.2%), and many lesions ulcerate (36.3%).
- After bleeding and crusting, the pyogenic granuloma can become smaller, but it usually regrows.
- The mean age of onset is 6.7 years; only 12.4% develop during the first year of life.
- Presentation is inversely correlated with age: younger than 5 years (42.1%), 5 to 10 years (30.4%), 10 to 15 years (23.0%), and 15 to 20 years (4.5%).
- A pyogenic granuloma involves the skin (88.2%) or mucous membranes (11.8%).
- Affects the head and neck (62%), trunk (20%), upper extremity (13%), or lower limb (5%).
- Head and neck lesions are most commonly located on the cheek (29%), oral cavity (14%), scalp (11%), forehead (10%), eyelid (9%), or lips (9%).
- 25% of patients have a history of trauma or an underlying cutaneous condition (such as capillary malformation or arteriovenous malformation).

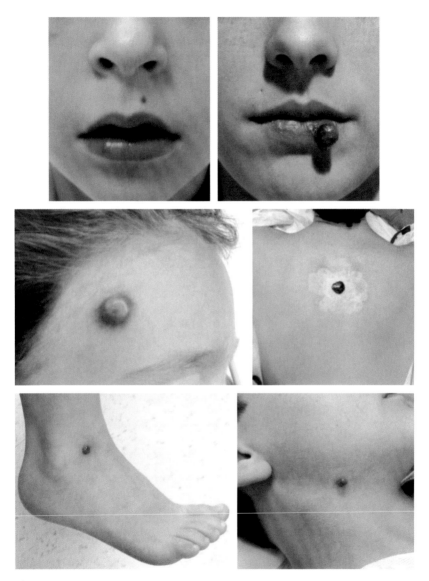

Fig. 6-1   Appearance of pyogenic granuloma. Lesions can be small, large, sessile, or pedunculated.

ETIOPATHOGENESIS

- Transcriptional profiling of laser-captured vessels from a pyogenic granuloma shows genes upregulated in the nitric oxide, hypoxia, and angiogenesis pathways.
- FLT4, a receptor related to pathologic angiogenesis, is specifically expressed.
- The current theory is that a pyogenic granuloma is a reactive lesion secondary to tissue injury. Wound healing is impaired and is driven by FLT4 and the nitric oxide pathway.

DIAGNOSIS

History and Physical Examination

- Diagnosis is made by history and physical examination. Imaging is unnecessary.
- A small red, bleeding lesion that presents during childhood is pathognomonic.
- Unlike other vascular tumors (infantile hemangioma, congenital hemangioma, kaposiform hemangioendothelioma), pyogenic granuloma is smaller, rarely present during the first month of life, and frequently bleeds.

Histopathology

- On low-power magnification, a pyogenic granuloma appears as an exophytic mass attached to a narrow stalk. It is superficial and shows immature capillaries with interspersed fibroblastic tissue resembling granulation in an edematous matrix.
- High-power magnification shows a polypoid dermal lesion with lobules of thin-walled capillaries with plump endothelial cells. Lesions usually involve the reticular dermis. The stroma has edema, fibrosis, and occasional inflammatory cells. The epithelium is atrophic, often ulcerated, and may have granulation tissue as well as lateral collarettes.

- A feeding artery is usually present at the base of the lesion. A normal number of mast cells is present, in contrast to a proliferating infantile hemangioma.
- A pyogenic granuloma is distinguished from an infantile hemangioma by its curved channels, intervascular stroma, and epidermal collarettes. Pyogenic granuloma also does not immunostain for GLUT1.

MANAGEMENT

- Although a pyogenic granuloma can rarely resolve spontaneously after it bleeds or ulcerates, lesions should not be observed. Pyogenic granuloma requires treatment to:
  - Prevent bleeding and ulceration
  - Improve a visible deformity
- Many treatment modalities have been described, such as resection, cautery, cryotherapy, curettage, shave excision, laser, and imiquimod cream.
- Because pyogenic granuloma usually involves the reticular dermis, definitive management is full-thickness skin excision (Fig. 6-2).

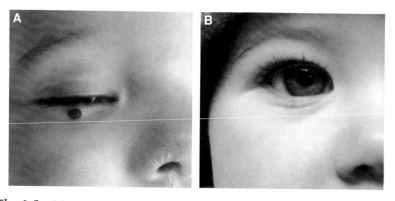

Fig. 6-2   Management of pyogenic granuloma. **A,** A 7-month-old girl with a 4-week history of an enlarging pyogenic granuloma of the lower eyelid. **B,** Three weeks postoperatively.

The recurrence rate after resection is less than 1%. Additional advantages of resection are that only one procedure is necessary, and the lesion can be sent for histopathologic analysis.
• Treatment methods other than full-thickness skin excision may not reach the deep component of the lesion and thus have a recurrence rate as high as 43%. Some methods (such as cryotherapy or laser) may require multiple procedures to achieve a cure and obviate the ability to send the lesion for histopathologic analysis.

Selected References

Godfraind C, Calicchio M, Kozakewich H. Pyogenic granuloma, an impaired wound healing process, linked to vascular growth driven by FLT4 and the nitric oxide pathway. Mod Pathol (in press).

Greene AK. Management of hemangiomas and other vascular tumors. Clin Plast Surg 38:45-63, 2011.

Gupta A, Kozakewich H. Histopathology of vascular anomalies. Clin Plast Surg 38:31-44, 2011.

Lee J, Sinno H, Tahiri Y, Gilardino MS. Treatment options for cutaneous pyogenic granulomas: a review. J Plast Reconstr Aesthet Surg 64:1216-1220, 2011.

Mills SE, Cooper PH, Fechner RE. Lobular capillary hemangioma: the underlying lesion of pyogenic granuloma. A study of 73 cases from the oral and nasal mucous membranes. Am J Surg Pathol 4:470-479, 1980.

Patrice SJ, Wiss K, Mulliken JB. Pyogenic granuloma (lobular capillary hemangioma): a clinicopathologic study of 178 cases. Pediatr Dermatol 8:267-276, 1991.

CHAPTER 7

Rare Vascular Tumors

TUMORS	MALFORMATIONS		
	Slow-Flow	**Fast-Flow**	**Overgrowth Syndromes**
Infantile Hemangioma	*Capillary Malformation*	*Arteriovenous Malformation*	CLOVES Klippel-Trenaunay Maffucci Parkes Weber Proteus Sturge-Weber
Congenital Hemangioma	*Lymphatic Malformation*		
Kaposiform Hemangioendothelioma	*Venous Malformation*		
Pyogenic Granuloma			
Rare Vascular Tumors Angiosarcoma Cutaneovisceral angiomatosis with thrombocytopenia Enzinger intramuscular hemangioma Epithelioid hemangioendothelioma Infantile myofibroma Tufted angioma			

ANGIOSARCOMA

- Angiosarcoma is an uncommon malignant tumor that constitutes less than 1% of soft tissue sarcomas.
- Approximately 99% of angiosarcomas affect adults, typically during the seventh decade of life. Usually sun-exposed areas of the head and neck are involved. The malignancy can occur in sites of previous radiation or in areas with long-standing lymphedema.
- Angiosarcoma is extremely rare in the pediatric population (approximately 1% of angiosarcomas). Males and females are affected equally, and the median age at diagnosis is 11 years.
- Pediatric tumors are located in the mediastinum (including heart and pericardium) (46%), liver (13%), breast (13%), spleen (7%), mesentery (7%), pelvis (7%), and upper limb (7%).
- Mean tumor size is 8 cm (range 3.5 to 13 cm).
- Histopathologically, two architectural patterns are seen: racemose vessels infiltrating normal tissue, and/or solid sheets or nests of cells.
- Areas of spindled or epithelioid malignant endothelial cells are present. Necrosis and significant cytologic atypia are visualized. Tumors have a high mitotic index (median 11 per 10 high-power fields).
- Treatment modalities include resection, radiation, and/or chemotherapy.
- Metastasis is common (usually to regional lymph nodes, lung, and liver), and mortality is 67%.

CUTANEOVISCERAL ANGIOMATOSIS WITH THROMBOCYTOPENIA (CAT)

- This disorder is also called *multifocal lymphangioendotheliomatosis with thrombocytopenia*.
- Multifocal vascular lesions occur that affect the skin and gastro-intestinal tract with thrombocytopenia (Fig. 7-1).
- The lung, bone, liver, spleen, and muscle also can be affected.
- Cutaneous lesions are noted at birth and appear reddish-brown with blue macules and papules.
- They primarily affect the trunk and extremities and are usually 5 mm or less in diameter. However, a dominant plaque several centimeters in size and large macules/plaques can occur.
- Some lesions (especially in the lungs) may exhibit postnatal growth.
- Patients develop hematemesis and/or melena. Endoscopy shows multifocal (as many as 100) mucosal lesions affecting all levels of the gastrointestinal tract (they measure between 1 and 10 mm).

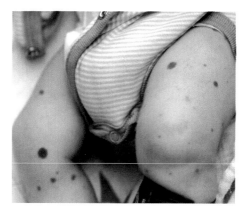

Fig. 7-1 A 2-month-old boy with cutaneovisceral angiomatosis with thrombocytopenia. Skin lesions were noted at birth, and the patient had thrombocytopenia, anemia, and gastrointestinal bleeding.

- Pulmonary involvement can cause hemoptysis.
- Histopathology shows thin-walled, blood-filled vessels with endothelial hyperplasia. Periodic acid–Schiff deposits are often present in the cytoplasm, and extracellular areas of endothelial hyperplasia are present. Lesions are negative for GLUT1. The endothelial proliferative index varies from 1% to 20%. Platelets are small, suggesting a primary defect in platelet function.
- The differential diagnosis includes hemangiomatosis, lymphangiomatosis, and blue rubber bleb nevus syndrome.
- MRI shows hyperintensity on T2 images and enhancement with contrast.
- Thrombocytopenia is diagnosed within the first 2 years of life, and platelet counts range from 50,000 to 100,000 mm^3. Platelet levels can decrease to 6000 mm^3 during disease exacerbation or periods of stress (such as infection or an operation).
- Platelets are small, serum fibrinogen is normal, and D-dimers are not present. A bone marrow biopsy shows megakaryocytic hyperplasia.
- Systemic antiangiogenic pharmacotherapy effectively reduces hemorrhage and the size of the lesions. Drugs that have been used successfully include corticosteroid, interferon, thalidomide, and vincristine.

ENZINGER INTRAMUSCULAR HEMANGIOMA

- Enzinger intramuscular hemangioma is also called *Enzinger hemangioma, small vessel type,* or *intramuscular hemangioma, capillary type.*
- It is a benign vascular tumor of skeletal muscle (Fig. 7-2).
- 25% are present in the pediatric age group. The median age at the time of diagnosis is 25 years.
- This affects the trunk (32%), head and neck (30%), upper limb (23%), or lower extremity (15%).

- The primary differential diagnosis is arteriovenous malformation, epithelioid hemangioendothelioma, infantile/congenital hemangioma, and infantile myofibroma.
- The tumor presents as a painless soft tissue swelling without overlying skin changes.
- Imaging findings are consistent with a tumor. The lesion shows fast-flow and enhancement.
- A biopsy is required for diagnosis.
- Histopathologically, the tumor is unencapsulated and can extend into subcutaneous fat and dermis. Aggregates or lobules of small, capillary-like vessels with plump endothelium and pericytes are separated by collagen. Lobules with enlarged capillaries can form a sinusoidal network that may drain into wide channels. Veins are often enlarged, and some have intimal or mural myofibroblastic cushions. Vessels infiltrate among muscle fibers and are accompanied by adipose tissue. Mitotic figures, plump nuclei, and perineural infiltration are common.
- Treatment is embolization and/or resection for symptomatic lesions. There is a 20% recurrence rate after excision.

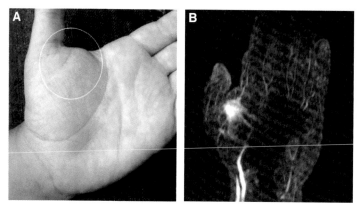

Fig. 7-2 **A,** A 6-year-old boy with a biopsy-proven Enzinger intramuscular hemangioma of the thenar area of the hand. **B,** MR image shows postcontrast enhancement of the lesion.

EPITHELIOID HEMANGIOENDOTHELIOMA (EHE)

- An epithelioid hemangioendothelioma is a malignant endothelial tumor with an unpredictable clinical course (Fig. 7-3).
- 7% occur in the pediatric population.
- The lesion is typically multifocal, affecting the skin, bone, liver, and lung (although other sites can be involved).
- Histologically, epithelioid endothelial cells appear round or polygonal and have an eosinophilic hyaline cytoplasm. Cytoplasmic vacuoles, usually containing erythrocytes, are present. Vesicular nuclei and inconspicuous nucleoli are common features. Most tumors appear infiltrative and have nests, cords, and short strands of epithelioid round or fusiform tumor cells. Angiocentric growth is often present, causing vessel occlusion and infiltration of vessel walls. Myxohyaline stroma shows degeneration, with hemorrhage and hemosiderin. Tumors stain for endothelial markers (CD31, CD34, factor VIII, UEA-1). Metaplastic bone is occasionally found.
- 70% of lesions have fewer than two mitoses per 10 high-power fields, but some tumors have more than six mitoses per 10 high-power fields. No correlation exists between nuclear atypia or mitoses and clinical behavior.
- Epithelioid hemangioendothelioma may remain stable, grow slowly, or progress rapidly, causing metastases (30%) and death (20%).
- Treatment is based on the clinical behavior of the tumor, and serial imaging is obtained. If minimal or no growth is noted, treatment is not mandatory. Enlarging or symptomatic lesions can be managed with systemic chemotherapy, resection, and/or radiation.
- Liver disease has been successfully treated with liver transplantation.

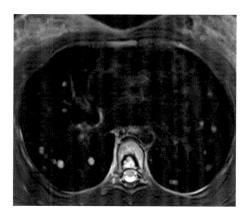

Fig. 7-3   Epithelioid hemangioendothelioma. Axial T2 MR sequence shows multiple lesions in the lung of a 15-year-old girl. Diagnosis was confirmed by histopathology.

INFANTILE MYOFIBROMA (IM)

- Infantile myofibroma was previously called *infantile hemangiopericytoma*.
- This is the most common benign fibrous tumor of infancy.
- There are three forms: (1) solitary (most common), (2) multifocal (infantile myofibromatosis), and (3) generalized (the viscera are affected).
- 60% are present at birth, and 80% are diagnosed before 2 years of age. Lesions can grow during infancy.
- Males are affected more often than females (1.6:1).
- Most commonly involves the head/neck, followed by the trunk and extremities.
- Infantile myofibromas can measure 0.5 to 7.0 cm and are typically located in the skin and subcutaneous tissue. Muscle, bone, or viscera are rarely affected.
- Cutaneous lesions can appear reddish-purple and may ulcerate. Subcutaneous nodules are typically rubbery and mobile.

- Infantile myofibroma can be difficult to diagnose clinically. The tumor is often mistaken for infantile or congenital hemangioma. Other lesions in the differential diagnosis include lymphatic malformation, infantile fibrosarcoma, and teratoma.
- Handheld Doppler probe examination exhibits fast-flow.
- Ultrasound illustrates a well-defined rim, thick septa, and vessels within an anechoic center.
- MRI shows hypointensity/isointensity on T1 sequences with peripheral enhancement after a contrast medium is administered. Lesions are hyperintense on T2 images, although the center may appear hypointense.
- Histopathologic evaluation is often necessary for diagnosis. Lesions have eosinophilic myofibroblasts in nodules, whorls, and/or fascicles, surrounded by poorly differentiated spindle cells with hyperchromatic nuclei. Central necrosis is common, with branching staghorn-shaped vessels surrounded by less-differentiated cells. Intravascular growth, mitotic figures, and hemangiopericytoma-like vessels are present. Immunostaining is positive for vimentin and smooth muscle actin. Tumors do not stain for S100 or desmin.
- Solitary infantile myofibroma can regress (30% to 60%) and thus lesions may be observed (Fig. 7-4). Resection is indicated for symptomatic tumors or to obtain a histopathologic diagnosis. A biopsy is often obtained, because it is difficult to accurately diagnose the lesions based on history, physical examination, and imaging.
- Multifocal infantile myofibromatosis has a favorable prognosis if the viscera are not involved. Management of lesions is similar to that for isolated infantile myofibroma.
- 25% to 40% of patients with multicentric infantile myofibromatosis will have visceral involvement (generalized myofibromatosis). The heart, lungs, gastrointestinal tract, and pancreas are most commonly affected. The mortality rate is 75%, and treatment of visceral lesions includes resection, chemotherapy, and/or radiation.

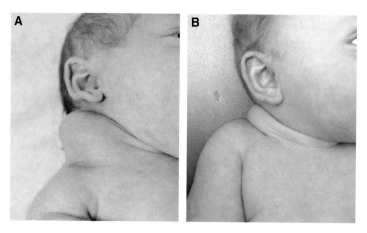

Fig. 7-4   A, A 2-week-old with biopsy-proven infantile myofibroma. **B,** Note the regression of the infantile myofibroma at 6 months of age.

TUFTED ANGIOMA (TA)

- Tufted angioma has been called *angioblastoma of Nakagawa* (Fig. 7-5).
- This tumor shares clinical and histopathologic features with kaposiform hemangioendothelioma but is less aggressive.
- The lesion can be locally invasive but does not metastasize.
- Tufted angioma presents during infancy and early childhood.
- Like kaposiform hemangioendothelioma, tufted angioma can be associated with Kasabach-Merritt phenomenon.
- Its appearance may be heterogenous: a solitary tumor, a diffuse stain, or a violaceous plaque.
- It most commonly appears as a pink-red plaque affecting the trunk or neck in young children.
- Histopathology shows round vascular nodules in the dermis or subcutis that are called *cannonballs*. The lobules contain well-defined capillaries with cuboidal plump endothelial cells. Spindled endothelial or mural cells may be present and immunostain for the lymphatic markers D240 and PROX1.

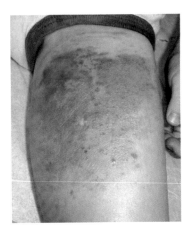

Fig. 7-5   A tufted angioma in a 2½-year-old boy. The painful lesion was noted at birth, and Kasabach-Merritt phenomenon was not present. The biopsy results were consistent with tufted angioma and he was treated with a corticosteroid followed by sirolimus.

- Tufted angioma is distinguished from kaposiform hemangioendothelioma by the small tufts of capillaries ("cannonballs") in the middle to lower third of the dermis.
- Asymptomatic tufted angiomas without Kasabach-Merritt phenomenon can be observed. Regression of some lesions has been reported.
- Symptomatic tumors may be excised if they are localized.
- Diffuse, unresectable lesions causing pain or Kasabach-Merritt phenomenon are treated with systemic pharmacotherapy. Vincristine is the first-line therapy, and sirolimus also may be effective. Second-line drugs include corticosteroid and interferon.
- Recently, low-dose aspirin has been shown to effectively reduce the size and symptoms of tufted angioma. Pulsed-dye laser and intense pulsed light also have been used to treat the tumor.

Selected References

Allen PW, Enzinger FM. Hemangioma of skeletal muscle: an analysis of 89 cases. Cancer 29:8-22, 1972.

Deyrup AT, Miettinen M, North PE, Khoury JD, Tighiouart M, Spunt SL, Parham D, Weiss SW, Shehata BM. Angiosarcomas arising in the viscera and soft tissue of children and young adults: a clinicopathologic study of 15 cases. Am J Surg Pathol 33:264-269, 2009.

Frieden IJ, Javvaji S. Response of tufted angiomas to low-dose aspirin. Pediatr Dermatol (in press).

Gupta A, Kozakewich H. Histopathology of vascular anomalies. Clin Plast Surg 38:31-44, 2011.

Jones EW, Orkin M. Tufted angioma (angioblastoma): a benign progressive angioma, not to be confused with Kaposi's sarcoma or low-grade angiosarcoma. J Am Acad Dermatol 20:214-225, 1989.

Mentzel T, Beham A, Calonje E, Katenkamp D, Fletcher C. Epithelioid hemangioendothelioma of skin and soft tissue: clinicopathologic and immunohistochemical study of 30 cases. Am J Surg Pathol 21:363-374, 1997.

Merrell SC, Rahbar R, Alomari AI, Padua HM, Vargas SO, Neufeld EJ, Dearden JL, Mulliken JB, Greene AK. Infantile myofibroma or lymphatic malformation: differential diagnosis of neonatal cystic cervicofacial lesions. J Craniofac Surg 21:422-426, 2010.

Weiss SW, Enzinger FM. Epithelioid hemangioendothelioma. A vascular tumor often mistaken for a carcinoma. Cancer 50:970-981, 1982.

Weiss SW, Goldblum JR. Benign tumors and tumor-like lesions of blood vessels. In Weiss SW, Goldblum JR, eds. Enzinger & Weiss's Soft Tissue Tumors, ed 5. St Louis: Elsevier-Mosby, 2008.

Vascular Malformations

III

TUMORS	MALFORMATIONS		
	Slow-Flow	**Fast-Flow**	**Overgrowth Syndromes**
Infantile Hemangioma	**Capillary Malformation** CLAPO Cutis marmorata Cutis marmorata telangiectatica congenita Diffuse capillary malformation with overgrowth Fading capillary stain Heterotopic neural nodule Macrocephaly–capillary malformation	**Arteriovenous Malformation** Capillary malformation–arteriovenous malformation Hereditary hemorrhagic telangiectasia *PTEN*-associated vascular anomaly Wyburn-Mason syndrome	CLOVES Klippel-Trenaunay Maffucci Parkes Weber Proteus Sturge-Weber
Congenital Hemangioma	**Lymphatic Malformation** Macrocystic Microcystic Combined (macrocystic/microcystic) Primary lymphedema Gorham-Stout disease Generalized lymphatic anomaly Kaposiform lymphangiomatosis		
Kaposiform Hemangioendothelioma	**Venous Malformation** Blue rubber bleb nevus syndrome Cerebral cavernous malformation Cutaneomucosal venous malformation Diffuse phlebectasia of Bockenheimer Fibroadipose vascular anomaly Glomuvenous malformation Phlebectasia Sinus pericranii Verrucous venous malformation		
Pyogenic Granuloma			
Rare Vascular Tumors			

CHAPTER 8

Capillary Malformation

TUMORS	MALFORMATIONS		
	Slow-Flow	**Fast-Flow**	**Overgrowth Syndromes**
Infantile Hemangioma	**Capillary Malformation** CLAPO Cutis marmorata Cutis marmorata telangiectatica congenita Diffuse capillary malformation with overgrowth Fading capillary stain Heterotopic neural nodule Macrocephaly–capillary malformation	***Arteriovenous Malformation***	CLOVES Klippel-Trenaunay Maffucci Parkes Weber Proteus Sturge-Weber
Congenital Hemangioma	**Lymphatic Malformation**		
Kaposiform Hemangioendothelioma	**Venous Malformation**		
Pyogenic Granuloma			
Rare Vascular Tumors			

CLINICAL FEATURES

- Capillary malformation (CM) was previously called *port-wine stain*.
- It is the most common type of vascular malformation, affecting 0.3% of newborns.
- Capillary malformation is present at birth and can involve any area of the integument.
- Males and females are affected equally.
- A capillary malformation may be localized, extensive, multiple, or generalized (for example, Sturge-Weber syndrome).
- The primary morbidity is psychosocial because of the pink-purple skin discoloration.
- Facial lesions often occur in a dermatomal distribution; 45% are restricted to one of the three trigeminal nerve distributions, while 55% overlap sensory dermatomes, cross the midline, or occur bilaterally.
- Over time, the lesion progresses:
  - It darkens and becomes more purple.
  - Fibrovascular cobblestoning can occur.
  - Pyogenic granulomas may develop in the lesion.
  - Soft tissue and bony overgrowth can occur underneath the area of the stain (Fig. 8-1).
- Capillary malformations affecting the trunk or extremity have less progression compared with lesions located on the face.
- When capillary malformation affects the face, 55% to 70% of patients have soft tissue hypertrophy (the lip is usually affected 81%); 22% to 45% have bony overgrowth (typically the maxilla, 83% to 94%); and 18% have localized cutaneous lesions (for example, pyogenic granulomas).
- Capillary malformations have several phenotypic variations (Fig. 8-2). Lesions can be syndromic and/or associated with underlying structural anomalies (Fig. 8-3).

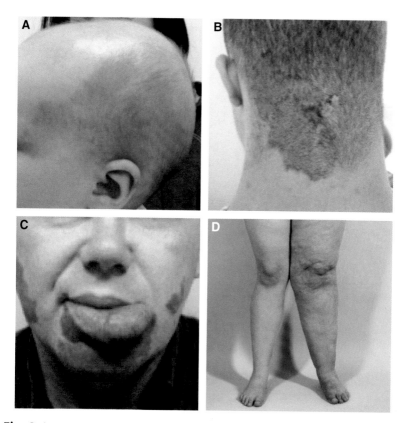

Fig. 8-1 Appearance of capillary malformations. **A,** Lesion affecting the forehead and scalp. Note the light appearance in infancy. **B,** Teenage boy with a capillary malformation of the posterior neck and scalp. It has darkened in color since infancy. Note the pyogenic granulomas located within the stain. **C,** Adult man with a facial capillary malformation causing soft tissue overgrowth of the lower lip. **D,** Adult woman with a diffuse capillary malformation with overgrowth (DCMO) of the left lower extremity.

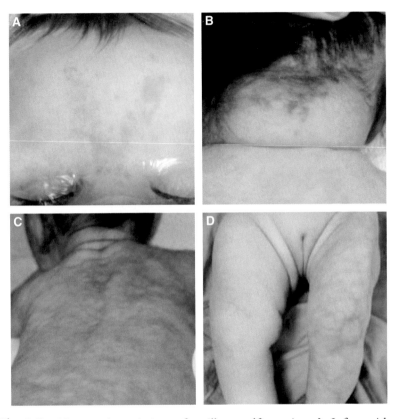

Fig. 8-2   Phenotypic variations of capillary malformation. **A,** Infant with a fading capillary stain of the forehead ("angel kiss"). **B,** Infant with a fading capillary stain of the posterior neck ("stork bite"). **C,** Cutis marmorata in a neonate. **D,** Cutis marmorata telangiectatica congenita of the lower extremity.

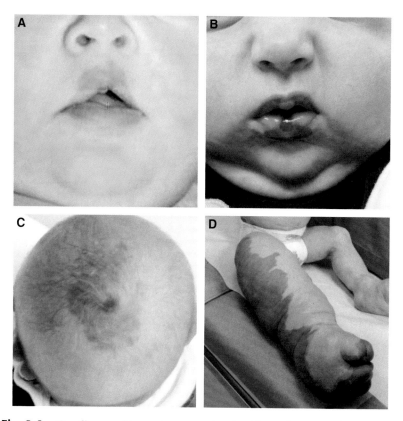

Fig. 8-3 Capillary malformations associated with syndromes and/or underlying anomalies. **A,** Infant female with macrocephaly–capillary malformation. Note stain involving the upper lip and philtrum. **B,** Infant with a CLAPO lesion of the lower lip. **C,** Heterotopic neural nodule. **D,** Lower extremity capillary malformation as a component of a combined vascular malformation syndrome.

ETIOPATHOGENESIS

- A defect in the developing nervous system might cause capillary malformation because (1) patterns are often regional or dermatomal (for example, trigeminal nerve distribution), (2) neuroectoderm contributes to the smooth muscle layers of vascular walls, (3) capillary malformations have decreased perivascular neural density, (4) abnormal innervation of leptomeningeal vessels can occur (Sturge-Weber syndrome), and (5) the cutaneous stain might result from the inability of blood vessels to constrict because of diminished sympathetic innervation.
- The cause of soft tissue and bony overgrowth beneath the stain is unknown. Progressive dilation of venules, angiogenesis, or vasculogenesis may contribute to the progression of capillary malformation.

PHENOTYPIC CONSIDERATIONS

Capillary Malformation of the Lower Lip, Lymphatic Malformation of the Face and Neck, Asymmetry, and Partial/Generalized Overgrowth (CLAPO)

- All affected patients have a capillary malformation of the lower lip that is pathognomonic for the condition.
- The capillary malformation is in the midline of the lower lip and is symmetrical, smooth, and well defined. Adjacent mucosal involvement is common.
- The lymphatic malformation component is typically microcystic and involves the oral cavity.
- Patients have normal cognitive development.
- Overgrowth can be localized or diffuse.

Cutis Marmorata

- An accentuated pattern of normal cutaneous vascularity is common in white infants.
- Transient mottling occurs in a low-temperature environment that disappears on warming.
- This is not a dermatopathologic condition.

Cutis Marmorata Telangiectatica Congenita (CMTC)

- Cutaneous marbling is present at birth, with an equal sex distribution.
- The skin is depressed, purple, and has a serpiginous, reticulated pattern.
- The lesion becomes more pronounced with lower temperatures.
- Ulceration is common.
- The condition is typically unilateral and may be localized, segmental, or generalized.
- CMTC usually affects the trunk or extremities. The lower limb is most commonly involved (69%).
- The affected extremity is often hypoplastic, and iliac or femoral stenosis can occur.
- Improvement occurs during the first year of life and can continue into adolescence.
- Atrophy, pigmentation, and ectasia of the superficial veins often persist.
- The differential diagnosis includes capillary malformation, cutis marmorata, and reticular hemangioma.

Diffuse Capillary Malformation With Overgrowth (DCMO)

- An extremity capillary malformation that causes soft tissue and often bony overgrowth of the limb.
- The lower extremity is more commonly affected than the upper limb.
- The extremity has increased circumference and may have axial overgrowth.
- An orthopedic consultation is obtained to assess for a leg-length discrepancy. A shoe-lift or epiphysiodesis may be necessary. Rarely, toe amputation is required so the patient can fit into shoes.
- Circumferential soft tissue overgrowth can cause:
  - Psychosocial morbidity because of limb asymmetry
  - Difficulty wearing clothing
- The cutaneous stain may be lightened using a pulsed-dye laser.
- Soft tissue overgrowth can be improved using suction-assisted lipectomy.

Fading Capillary Stain

- A fading capillary stain is the most common vascular birthmark, present in 50% of white newborns.
- Has been called an "angel kiss" if located on the forehead, eyelids, nose, or upper lip.
- When it is present on the posterior neck, it has been called a "stork bite."
- No treatment is necessary, because it lightens over the first 2 years of life.
- If a residual lesion causes psychosocial morbidity, it can be treated with a pulsed-dye laser.

Heterotopic Neural Nodule

- A heterotopic neural nodule is a parietal or occipital scalp nodule with overlying alopecia, a surrounding capillary malformation, and a ring of long hair ("hair collar sign").
- Lesions contain heterotopic leptomeningeal (and occasionally glial) tissue.
- 50% of heterotopic neural nodules extend intracranially.
- An MRI is obtained to determine whether a connection to the dura exists.
- Management is by resection. A neurosurgical consultation is obtained if preoperative imaging shows dural involvement.

Macrocephaly–Capillary Malformation (M-CM)

- Patients with M-CM have macrocephaly (>95th percentile), developmental delay, a capillary malformation involving the philtrum/upper lip (approximately 75%), and a diffuse capillary malformation involving the trunk or extremities.
- The trunk or extremity stain is a patchy, reticular capillary malformation (not cutis marmorata telangiectatica congenita or cutis marmorata).
- Unlike cutis marmorata telangiectatica congenita, the lesion does not ulcerate or fade, and the lower limb is often hypertrophied.
- Neurologic abnormalities are common (developmental delay, megalencephaly, hydrocephalus).

DIAGNOSIS

History and Physical Examination

- Diagnosis of a capillary malformation is made by history and physical examination. Imaging and histopathology are unnecessary.
- Lesions affect the skin, are present at birth, and slowly darken.
- Fast-flow is not present on handheld Doppler examination.

Imaging

- Radiographic studies are not diagnostic for capillary malformation.
- Ultrasonography and MRI may show thickened skin, with dilated cutaneous or subcutaneous veins and increased subcutaneous adipose tissue.
- An MRI is obtained preoperatively for patients who have problematic soft tissue overgrowth underneath the capillary malformation. If a significant amount of subcutaneous adipose tissue is present, patients may benefit from suction-assisted lipectomy.
- CT is used to assess bony overgrowth underneath the stain if operative intervention is planned.

Histopathology

- Capillary malformation is diagnosed by history and physical examination; a biopsy is rarely indicated.
- In young children, the papillary dermis contains dilated capillaries with thin walls and narrow lumens.
- As the child ages, vessel size and density increase. Ectatic, venule-like vessels become more prominent in the papillary and reticular dermis. Vessels contain flat endothelial cells, thin walls, and a layer of pericytes. Intervascular fibrous tissue increases.

- Over time, vessel size and area continue to increase. Cutaneous thickening and nodules correlate with enlarged veins that extend into the reticular dermis and subcutis. Vessels have thickened walls and are surrounded by fibrous tissue. The epidermis and dermal appendages become hyperplastic.

MANAGEMENT

Pulsed-Dye Laser (595 nm Wavelength)

- Treatment with a pulsed-dye laser improves the appearance of capillary malformation by lightening its color (Fig. 8-4).
- The laser penetrates only 0.75 to 1.2 mm into the dermis and thus deeper or larger vessels may not be affected.
- The settings used are pulse duration (0.45 to 1.5 ms), fluence (6 to 10 J/cm^2), and spot size (7 to 10 mm).

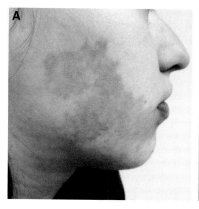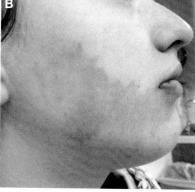

Fig. 8-4   Management of capillary malformation using pulsed-dye laser. **A,** A 20-year-old woman with a capillary malformation involving the right side of the face. **B,** Lightened appearance of the lesion after two treatments. (Photos courtesy of Sheilagh Maguiness, MD.)

- Intervention during infancy or early childhood is recommended (especially if the malformation is located on the face) because superior lightening of the lesion is achieved, the risk of darkening and hypertrophy is reduced, and psychosocial morbidity is minimized.
- The head and neck area responds better to laser treatment than the extremities do.
- The outcome is superior for smaller lesions and those treated at a younger age.
- 15% of patients achieve at least 90% lightening, 65% improve 50% to 90%, and 20% respond poorly.
- The efficacy of pulsed-dye laser treatment is inferior for Asian patients; only 14% show 50% or more lightening.
- Pigmentary changes and scarring are more likely to affect individuals with darker skin.
- After treatment, capillary malformation usually redarkens over time, and patients benefit from repeat intervention.
- Infants can be treated while awake (using a topical anesthetic), depending on the size and location of the capillary malformation. After infancy, it is more difficult to restrain a child, and general anesthesia is preferred, unless the lesion is small. Adolescents generally tolerate laser treatment while awake, depending on the location and extent of the capillary malformation.
- Multiple treatments, spaced 6 weeks apart, are often required until no further improvement is evident.
- Some families may elect to wait to treat a capillary malformation of the trunk or extremities until the child is old enough to make the decision.
- If the capillary malformation is light, patients or families may postpone laser therapy until the lesion darkens and becomes more visible.

- Following laser treatment, reactivation of herpes simplex virus, superinfection of molluscum contagiosum, and/or development of warts can occur.
- Pulsed-dye laser treatment is less effective for capillary malformations that have progressed to a dark color with cutaneous thickening and/or cobblestoning.

Operative Treatment

- Capillary malformations typically do not require operative intervention.
- Surgical procedures are not indicated to remove the cutaneous stain, but rather to correct overgrowth caused by the malformation (for example, pyogenic granulomas, fibrovascular nodules, and soft tissue or osseous hypertrophy) (Fig. 8-5).

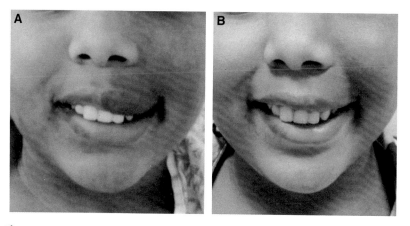

Fig. 8-5 Operative management of capillary malformation. **A,** A 13-year-old girl with a capillary malformation of the upper lip and cheek causing labial overgrowth. **B,** Improved lip contour 2½ months after transverse mucosal excision of hypertrophied tissue.

- Because overgrowth is not present at birth, patients do not typically require operative intervention until adolescence or adulthood.
- Patients with facial lesions causing soft tissue or bony overgrowth undergo labial reduction (61%), excision of localized cutaneous growths (33%), malar contouring (11%), palpebral debulking (11.0%), and/or orthognathic correction (11%).
- Small fibrovascular nodules or pyogenic granulomas can be excised.
- A trunk or extremity capillary malformation associated with increased subcutaneous adipose tissue can be improved with suction-assisted lipectomy.
- Severe cutaneous thickening and cobblestoning may be resected and reconstructed by linear closure, skin grafts, or local flaps.
- Facial asymmetry caused by overgrowth of the zygoma, maxilla, or mandible can be improved by contour burring.
- Enlargement of the maxilla or mandible may result in an occlusal cant (vertical maxillary overgrowth), with increased dental show and malocclusion. Malocclusion is addressed in adolescence with orthodontic management. If correction of the occlusion cannot be achieved with orthodontics, an orthognathic procedure is considered after skeletal growth is complete (age 16 in girls and age 18 in boys). A LeFort I osteotomy or bimaxillary procedure may be necessary.

Selected References

Chapas AM, Eickhorst K, Geronemus RG. Efficacy of early treatment of facial port wine stains in newborns: a review of 49 cases. Lasers Surg Med 39:563-568, 2007.

Devillers AC, de Waard-van der Spek FB, Oranje AP. Cutis marmorata telangiectatica congenita: clinical features in 35 cases. Arch Dermatol 135:34-38, 1999.

Greene AK, Taber SF, Ball KL, Padwa BL, Mulliken JB. Sturge-Weber syndrome: frequency and morbidity of facial overgrowth. J Craniofac Surg 20:617-621, 2009.

Gupta A, Kozakewich H. Histopathology of vascular anomalies. Clin Plast Surg 38:31-44, 2011.

Huikeshoven M, Koster PH, de Borgie CA, Beek JF, van Gemert MJ, van der Horst CM. Redarkening of port-wine stains 10 years after pulsed-dye-laser treatment. N Engl J Med 356:1235-1240, 2007.

Maguiness SM, Liang MG. Management of capillary malformations. Clin Plast Surg 38:65-73, 2011.

Tan OT, Sherwood K, Gilchrest BA. Treatment of children with port-wine stains using the flashlamp-pulsed tunable dye laser. N Engl J Med 320:416-421, 1989.

Toriello HV, Mulliken JB. Accurately renaming macrocephaly-cutis marmorata telangiectatica congenital (M-CMTC) as macrocephaly-capillary malformation (M-CM). Am J Med Gen A 143A:3009, 2007.

van der Horst CM, Koster PH, de Borgie CA, Bossuyt PM, van Gemert MJ. Effect of the timing of treatment of port-wine stains with the flashlamp-pumped pulsed-dye laser. N Engl J Med 338:1028-1033, 1998.

Lymphatic Malformation

TUMORS	MALFORMATIONS		
	Slow-Flow	**Fast-Flow**	**Overgrowth Syndromes**
Infantile Hemangioma	*Capillary Malformation*	*Arteriovenous Malformation*	CLOVES Klippel- Trenaunay Maffucci Parkes Weber Proteus Sturge-Weber
Congenital Hemangioma	*Lymphatic Malformation* Macrocystic Microcystic Combined (macrocystic/ microcystic) Primary lymphedema Gorham-Stout disease Generalized lymphatic anomaly Kaposiform lymphangiomatosis		
Kaposiform Hemangioendothelioma	*Venous Malformation*		
Pyogenic Granuloma			
Rare Vascular Tumors			

CLINICAL FEATURES

- Lymphatic malformation (LM) is defined by the size of its channels (Fig. 9-1):
  - *Macrocystic* (cysts large enough to be treated by sclerotherapy)
  - *Microcystic* (cysts too small to be cannulated by a needle)
  - *Combined* (macrocystic/microcystic)
- Lesions are usually noted at birth, although small or deep lymphatic malformations may not become evident until childhood or adolescence, after they have enlarged and/or become symptomatic.
- Lymphatic malformations are soft and compressible. The overlying skin may be normal, have a bluish hue, or contain pink vesicles that can appear similar to a capillary malformation.
- The most commonly affected sites are the head and neck and axilla.
- Because the lymphatic and venous systems share a common embryologic origin, lymphatic malformations may be associated with venous phlebectasia (previously called *lymphatic-venous malformation*).
- Lymphatic malformation causes three primary problems: (1) psychosocial morbidity, because lesions typically involve the integument and cause a deformity, (2) infection, and (3) bleeding.
- Swelling from bleeding, infection, or a viral illness may obstruct vital structures.
- Infection occurs because malformed lymphatics are unable to normally clear foreign material and contribute to antibody production, and proteinaceous fluid and blood in the cysts favor bacterial growth.
- 71% of lesions become infected, and sepsis can occur rapidly. Poor dental hygiene predisposes cervicofacial malformations to infection, and buttock or pelvic lesions may become infected by gut flora.

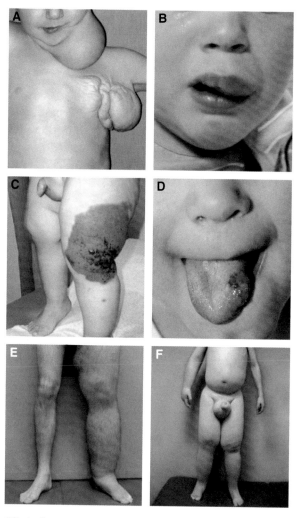

Fig. 9-1 Clinical presentation of lymphatic malformation. **A,** Macrocystic lymphatic malformation of the neck and axilla. **B,** Microcystic lymphatic malformation affecting the upper lip. **C,** Cutaneous microcystic lymphatic malformation with bleeding and draining vesicles. **D,** Intraoral microcystic lymphatic malformation with vesicles on the tongue. **E,** Primary lymphedema of the left lower extremity. **F,** Generalized lymphatic anomaly (GLA) causing lymphedema of three extremities and the scrotum, chylous pleural effusions, ascites, and malabsorption.

- Intralesional bleeding affects approximately one third of lymphatic malformations and causes bluish discoloration, pain, and/or swelling. Bleeding results from abnormal venous channels in the malformation or from small arteries in the septations.
- Lymphatic malformation can cause site-specific morbidity depending on the extent and location of the lesion:
  - Cutaneous vesicles may have malodorous drainage.
  - Oral lesions can lead to macroglossia, pain, poor hygiene, and caries.
  - Thoracic or abdominal lymphatic malformations may result in pleural, pericardial, or peritoneal chylous effusions.
  - Periorbital lesions can lead to proptosis (45%), ptosis (52%), amblyopia (33%), reduced vision (40%), and blindness (7%).
  - Intestinal lesions may cause malabsorption.
  - Cervicofacial lymphatic malformations often require tracheostomy to maintain the airway (67%).
  - Upper extremity lesions can limit function and affect the brachial plexus.
  - Osseous lymphatic malformations can cause either bone destruction or secondary bony overgrowth.
- Lymphatic malformations progress over time: 42% before adolescence, 85% before adulthood, and 95% over the patient's lifetime. Progression is 2.6 times more likely to occur in adolescence than in childhood. Consequently, most patients who present with asymptomatic lesions will ultimately require intervention.

ETIOPATHOGENESIS

- Theories for the formation of lymphatic malformations include:
  - Disruption of the lymph sacs during the sixth week of embryonic life.
  - Sprouting lymphatic channels become pinched off from the main lymphatic system, leading to aberrant collections of lymphatic fluid–filled spaces.

- Abnormal budding of the lymphatic system occurs, with a loss of connection to the central lymph channels.
- Lymphatic tissue develops in aberrant locations.
- Although a somatic mutation for lymphatic malformations has not been found, germline mutations can cause primary lymphedema (such as *VEGFR3, FOXC2, SOX18,* and *CCBE1*).
- The cause of progression of lymphatic malformations is unknown. Possible mechanisms might be dilation of vascular spaces, angiogenesis, lymphangiogenesis, or vasculogenesis. Because lesions have a higher risk of enlargement during adolescence, pubertal hormones may stimulate lymphatic malformations.

PHENOTYPIC CONSIDERATIONS

Macrocystic Lymphatic Malformation

- Macrocystic lesions contain cysts large enough to be accessed by a needle (typically 5 mm or larger), and thus are amenable to sclerotherapy.
- Most commonly the neck or axilla is affected.
- Macrocystic lymphatic malformations rarely can improve spontaneously.
- These lesions have a better prognosis than microcystic lymphatic malformations, because they can be treated with sclerotherapy.

Microcystic Lymphatic Malformation

- Microcystic lesions have cysts that are too small to be cannulated by a needle (usually less than 5 mm), and thus cannot be treated by sclerotherapy.
- Most commonly these affect the face and extremities.
- Lesions are often associated with cutaneous vesicles that can bleed and leak lymphatic fluid.
- The prognosis is inferior to microcystic lymphatic malformations, because they are not amenable to sclerotherapy.

Combined (Macrocystic and Microcystic) Lymphatic Malformation

- Approximately half of lymphatic malformations are not purely macrocystic or microcystic; they contain both macrocysts and microcysts.
- The prognosis and treatment are based on the ratio of macrocystic to microcystic disease. The greater the macrocystic composition of the lesion, the better the prognosis, because most of the lesion can be treated with sclerotherapy. In contrast, a primarily microcystic lesion will only have minimal benefit from sclerotherapy to its minor macrocystic component.

Primary Lymphedema

- Primary lymphedema typically results from hypoplastic lymphatic development in an extremity.
- The condition usually presents in infancy or adolescence and most commonly involves the lower limb.
- Several germline mutations can cause primary lymphedema (such as *VEGFR3, FOXC2, SOX18,* and *CCBE1*).

Gorham–Stout Disease (GSD)

- Gorham-Stout disease is a progressive osseous lymphatic anomaly that causes osteolysis of bone. It is also called the *disappearing bone disease.*
- The mean number of involved bones is seven. If multiple sites are involved, they are contiguous.
- Males and females are affected equally.
- Over time, the bone resorbs and causes pain, pathologic fractures, and significant morbidity.
- Bony changes are characterized by progressive osteolysis with resorption and cortical loss.
- The ribs are most commonly affected, followed by the cranium, clavicle, and cervical spine.

- 95% of lesions have an associated infiltrative soft tissue abnormality at the site of bone involvement.
- 42% of patients develop pleural effusions, and 21% have splenic and/or hepatic lesions.
- Histopathology shows variably sized lymphatic channels in the medulla and cortex that are immunopositive for lymphatic markers (for example, D240).
- Management involves weekly subcutaneous interferon injection and monthly intravenous bisphosphonate therapy. This treatment regimen can prevent continued bone loss but rarely promotes remineralization. Sirolimus recently has been used to treat the disease.

Generalized Lymphatic Anomaly (GLA)

- Generalized lymphatic anomaly is a multisystem disorder affecting noncontiguous areas.
- The condition was previously called *lymphangiomatosis.*
- Males and females are affected equally.
- 85% of patients have bony involvement, and the mean number of affected bones is 30.
- In contrast to Gorham-Stout disease, osseous lesions show discrete lytic areas or radiolucencies confined to the medullary cavity. Although the number and size of lesions can increase over time, progressive osteolysis and cortical loss does not occur.
- The most commonly affected bone is a rib, followed by the thoracic spine, humerus, and femur. Bony involvement (88%) is more likely to involve the appendicular skeleton (the shoulders, pelvis, and upper and lower extremities), compared with Gorham-Stout disease (26%). Both Gorham-Stout disease and generalized lymphatic anomaly usually affect the axial skeleton (the cranium, facial bones, rib cage, sternum, and vertebral column).
- 56% of affected children have an associated infiltrative soft tissue abnormality adjacent to the area of bone involvement.

- 50% of patients have a macrocystic lymphatic malformation, 63% exhibit splenic or hepatic lesions, and 50% experience pleural effusions.
- Histopathologic findings are similar to those of Gorham-Stout disease (variably sized lymphatic channels in the medulla and cortex that are immunopositive for lymphatic markers). However, more new bone formation, greater marrow fibrosis, and increased osteoclastic/osteoblastic activity are exhibited in generalized lymphatic anomaly than in Gorham-Stout disease.
- If symptomatic bony destruction occurs, patients are given a weekly subcutaneous interferon injection and monthly intravenous bisphosphonates. This treatment regimen can prevent continued bone loss but rarely stimulates remineralization. Alternatively, sirolimus has shown favorable preliminary results.

Kaposiform Lymphangiomatosis (KLA)

- Kaposiform lymphangiomatosis is a variant of generalized lymphatic anomaly that causes thrombocytopenia and/or tissue hemorrhage.
- The male to female ratio is 2:1, and the mean age at which initial symptoms present is 8 years (range 1 year to 41 years).
- Patients most commonly present with cough or dyspnea (55%), and 85% develop pericardial and/or pleural effusions; 25% of patients have a cutaneous stain and/or nodule.
- Thrombocytopenia affects 30% of patients with a mean platelet count of 50,000 (range 20,000 to 69,000/µl).
- Kaposiform lymphangiomatosis involves the mediastinum (95%), bone (40%), spleen (35%), and/or retroperitoneum (30%).
- Treatment includes drainage of symptomatic effusions, pleurodesis, sclerotherapy, and medical therapy, such as corticosteroids, vincristine, thalidomide, and sirolimus.
- Although combination therapy can improve symptoms, the prognosis is poor and the mortality rate is high.
- Histopathologic examination shows abnormally dilated lymphatic channels, as seen with generalized lymphatic anomaly.

Solid or reticular clusters of parallel spindled, hemosiderotic, lymphatic endothelial cells are present. They are located intraluminally or paraluminally and contain erythrocytes and hemorrhage. Mitoses and cellular atypia is minimal.

DIAGNOSIS

History and Physical Examination

- 90% of lymphatic malformations are diagnosed by history and physical examination.
- The primary differential diagnosis is venous malformation.
- If the diagnosis is unclear after history-taking and physical examination, handheld Doppler examination will differentiate lymphatic malformation from fast-flow lesions (such as hemangioma and arteriovenous malformation).
- Small superficial lymphatic malformations do not require further diagnostic workup.

Imaging

- Large or deep lymphatic malformations are evaluated by MRI to confirm the diagnosis, define the type of malformation (macrocystic, microcystic, or combined), determine the extent of disease, and plan treatment (Fig. 9-2).
- MRI sequences are obtained with fat suppression and gadolinium to help differentiate lymphatic malformation from venous malformation. On T1 images cysts are hypointense. Following contrast administration, macrocystic lesions only show enhancement of the wall and septations (venous malformations have more diffuse, heterogeneous enhancement). Lymphatic malformations are more infiltrative than venous malformations. Lymphatic malformations appear as a cystic lesion (macrocystic, microcystic, or combined) with septations of variable thickness. Because lymphatic malformations have a high water content, they are hyperintense on T2 sequences (after treatment, fibrosis

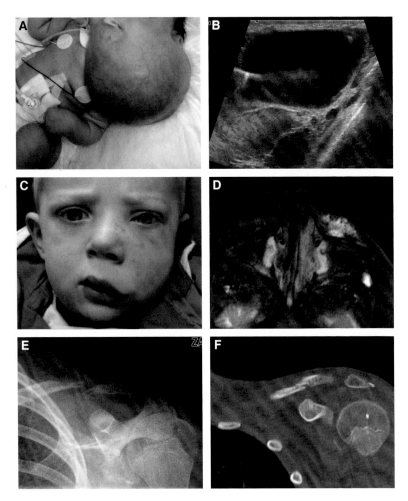

Fig. 9-2 Radiographic appearance of lymphatic malformation. Determining whether a lymphatic malformation is macrocystic or microcystic has important implications for treatment, because macrocysts are amenable to sclerotherapy. **A,** A male infant with a large macrocystic lymphatic malformation of the neck. **B,** Ultrasound shows anechoic macrocysts with echogenic intervening septa. **C,** A 2-year-old boy with a microcystic lymphatic malformation of the left side of his face. **D,** His T2 MRI shows a bright lesion primarily in the subcutaneous tissue without macrocysts. **E,** Plain radiograph and **F,** CT image of a 17-year-old boy with biopsy-proven Gorham-Stout disease causing progressive loss of the clavicle. He was treated with interferon and bisphosphonates.

causes lesions to become less hyperintense). Macrocystic lymphatic malformations often have fluid levels because of intracystic blood or proteinaceous fluid. Microcystic lesions are hypointense on T1 sequences and hyperintense on T2 images. The borders of microcystic lymphatic malformations are comparatively ill defined and have slightly greater enhancement, compared with macrocystic lesions.

- Ultrasonography is not as informative as MRI, but sedation in children is not required for ultrasound. An ultrasound can provide diagnostic confirmation, document intralesional bleeding, and differentiate between macrocystic and microcystic lesions. Macrocystic lymphatic malformations show anechoic cysts with thin echogenic septations, often with debris or fluid-fluid levels. Doppler studies demonstrate vessels within the septations. Microcystic lymphatic malformations have ill-defined, hyperechoic masses with diffuse involvement of adjacent tissues.
- CT scans and plain films are occasionally indicated to delineate osseous involvement, particularly if resection is planned.
- Lymphoscintigraphy is used to definitively diagnose primary lymphedema and determine the severity of lymphatic dysfunction.

Histopathology

- Histologic confirmation of a lymphatic malformation is rarely necessary, because lesions are diagnosed by history, physical examination, and imaging. A biopsy may be indicated if imaging is equivocal or if a malignant process is suspected.
- Macrocystic lymphatic malformations contain thick walls with myxoid fibrous tissue, myofibroblasts, and minimal smooth muscle.
- Microcystic lymphatic malformations have small, thin-walled lymphatic channels with flat endothelial cells without smooth

muscle. Lymphatic channels can contain eosinophilic protein-rich fluid with lymphocytes, macrophages, red blood cells, and/or hemosiderin.

- When the skin is involved, an expanded papillary dermis with thin-walled lymphatic channels is present. Verruciform hyperplasia and large lymphatic channels with thin muscular walls can be located in the reticular dermis. The dermis may also contain fibrous tissue as well as lymphoid collections, with germinal centers and plasma cells.

- Compared with a solitary lymphatic malformation, generalized lymphatic malformation exhibits smaller channels, larger lymphatic endothelial cells, endothelial hyperplasia, and an increased proliferative index.

- Lymphatic malformations immunostain for the lymphatic markers D240, LYVE1, and PROX1. Consequently, immunohistochemistry with these antibodies can be used to differentiate lymphatic malformations from other vascular anomalies.

MANAGEMENT

Nonoperative Treatment

- Lymphatic malformation is benign, and thus intervention is not mandatory. Small or asymptomatic lesions may be observed.

- Intralesional bleeding is treated conservatively with pain medication and occasionally prophylactic antibiotics because bleeding may predispose to infection.

- An infected lymphatic malformation often cannot be controlled with oral antibiotics, and intravenous antimicrobial therapy usually is required.

- Patients with more than three infections in a year are given daily prophylactic antibiotic therapy.

- Because a lymphatic malformation is at risk for infection, good oral hygiene should be maintained, and patients should avoid incidental trauma to the lesion.
- Recently oral pharmacotherapy using sirolimus has shown promising results for the treatment of severe microcystic lymphatic malformations.

Timing of Intervention

- Intervention for lymphatic malformation is reserved for symptomatic lesions (pain, significant deformity, or threatened vital structures) or for large, asymptomatic macrocystic lesions.
- Most children do not require treatment at the time of diagnosis. Because a lymphatic malformation slowly expands over time, patients may become symptomatic and seek intervention in childhood or adolescence.
- Less commonly, a lymphatic malformation involving an anatomically sensitive area or one that causes a deformity necessitates management as early as infancy. For example, a lesion obstructing the airway or visual axis requires urgent intervention.
- Asymptomatic macrocystic lesions are usually treated prophylactically with sclerotherapy before they bleed or become infected which can make the lesion microcystic and no longer amenable to sclerotherapy. If possible, intervention should be postponed until after the patient is 12 months of age, when the risks associated with anesthesia are lower.
- Intervention for a lesion causing a visible deformity should be considered before 4 years of age to limit psychological morbidity. At this age, long-term memory and self-esteem begin to form. Some parents may elect to wait until the child is older and able to make the decision to proceed with operative intervention, especially if the deformity is minor.

Sclerotherapy

- Sclerotherapy is the first-line mode of treatment for a large or problematic macrocystic or combined lymphatic malformation (Fig. 9-3).
- The procedure involves aspiration of the cysts, followed by injection of an inflammatory substance that causes scarring of the cyst walls to each other. Although sclerotherapy does not remove the lymphatic malformation, it effectively shrinks the lesion.
- The most commonly used sclerosants include doxycycline, sodium tetradecyl sulfate, ethanol, bleomycin, and OK-432 (killed group A *Streptococcus pyogenes*).
- Almost all macrocystic lymphatic malformations will have an excellent response to sclerotherapy. Improvement for combined lymphatic malformations is superior for lesions with a greater macrocystic composition. Microcystic lymphatic malformations do not respond to sclerotherapy (although bleomycin may have some efficacy).
- Sclerotherapy provides superior results and has lower morbidity compared with resection. It is four times more likely to be successful and has one tenth the complication rate. Long-term control of lymphatic malformation is favorable; 90% do not regrow 3 years after treatment.
- The preferred sclerosant at our institution is doxycycline, because it is very effective (83% reduction in size) and safe. Doxycycline also theoretically may prevent infectious complications. A solution of 10 mg/ml is injected, and up to 50 ml (500 mg) may be used for infants and small children. Older children and adults may be treated with as much as 100 ml (1000 mg). Sodium tetradecyl sulfate (STS) is our second-line sclerosant for lymphatic malformations.
- Bleomycin causes minimal swelling and is considered for lymphatic malformations in difficult anatomic areas such as the oral cavity or airway, or for lesions that have not been responsive to other agents. Bleomycin may have some benefit for microcystic lesions that are not amenable to resection.

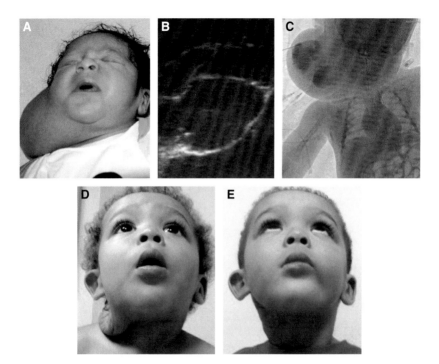

Fig. 9-3   Management of macrocystic lymphatic malformation. **A,** A male infant with a large lesion involving the neck. **B,** Ultrasound confirms the presence of macrocysts. **C,** Contrast injection of macrocysts during sclerotherapy. **D,** Two years after sclerotherapy, the child has residual skin excess. **E,** The boy is seen 7 months after resection of redundant skin.

- Ethanol is an effective sclerosant, but it has the highest complication rate. It can be used for small lesions, but large volumes should be avoided to reduce the risk of local and systemic toxicity. Ethanol can injure nerves and thus should not be used in proximity to important structures such as the facial nerve.
- OK-432 is not widely available, but it is an effective sclerosant; 94% of macrocystic lymphatic malformations and 63% of combined lesions will have a greater than 60% reduction in size with minimal morbidity.

- Small lesions in adolescents or adults may be treated in the office without image guidance; 3% sodium tetradecyl sulfate is diluted with saline to inject a 1% solution.
- Most patients, especially children, are managed under general anesthesia. Lesions are treated using ultrasound and/or fluoroscopic guidance.
- A contrast medium can be injected to determine the anatomy of complex lesions, but this is usually not performed. After fluid is aspirated from the cyst, the sclerosant is injected. Because lymphatic malformation is at risk for infection, patients are given periprocedural antibiotics.
- Large cysts occasionally require placement of a pigtail catheter and sequential drainage and injection over several days. Resolution of macrocysts may occur within days, but can take 6 to 8 weeks.
- Depending on the size of the lymphatic malformation, and whether there are residual macrocysts, additional injections every 6 to 8 weeks might be required.
- Posttreatment edema progresses for 24 to 48 hours. Except for young infants and individuals with airway lesions, most patients are discharged home on the day of the procedure. Posttreatment edema around the airway may necessitate monitoring in the intensive care unit, prolonged intubation, or a tracheostomy.
- Orbital injections can cause orbital compartment syndrome, so patients are examined by an ophthalmologist before and after sclerotherapy.
- Ulceration is the most common complication of sclerotherapy (less than 5% of cases). It is more likely with superficial lesions and when ethanol is used. Ulceration is managed using local wound care, and the area is allowed to heal secondarily.
- Systemic complications of sclerotherapy can occur when ethanol is used (doxycycline and sodium tetradecyl sulfate are not associated with significant systemic adverse effects). Ethanol may cause central nervous system depression, pulmonary hypertension, hemolysis, thromboembolism, and arrhythmias. Transient (5%) or permanent (2.5%) nerve injury can also occur after ethanol sclerotherapy.

- Lymphatic malformations may reexpand over time; 9% recur within 3 years after OK-432 treatment, and most will enlarge with longer follow-up. Consequently, patients often need repeat sclerotherapy over their lifetime. If a problematic lymphatic malformation recurs and macrocysts are not present, resection is the next treatment option.

Radiofrequency Ablation (RFA)

- For radiofrequency ablation, low-temperature tissue destruction is used, which limits thermal injury to the surrounding structures.
- This is the first-line intervention for problematic mucosal vesicles in the oral cavity.
- Compared with carbon dioxide laser treatment, patients recover faster and have less postoperative edema. Reduced swelling is preferable in the oral cavity, because patients can more easily resume feeding, and there is less risk of airway compromise.
- The low-frequency mode removes a superficial layer of tissue, and the high-frequency option destroys deeper tissue.
- Patients have minimal postoperative pain and may resume an oral diet within 24 hours of the procedure.
- In a study of 22 patients who underwent radiofrequency ablation, none required postprocedure intubation for swelling.

Operative Treatment

- Resection of a macrocystic lymphatic malformation generally is not indicated unless the lesion is symptomatic and sclerotherapy is no longer possible because all of the macrocysts have been treated, or excision may be curative because the lesion is small and well localized.
- Excision is usually subtotal, because lymphatic malformations typically involve multiple tissue planes and important structures. Consequently, recurrence is common (17% to 64%), and thus sclerotherapy is the preferred treatment for macrocystic or combined lesions.

- Nonproblematic microcystic malformations can be observed. Extirpation is reserved for symptomatic lesions because excision is usually subtotal, recurrence is common, a scar is placed in the area of the malformation, and the patient can have complications from the procedure, such as bleeding, infection, wound healing problems, or poor scarring.
- Bleomycin sclerotherapy is often attempted before resection of a microcystic lesion in an unfavorable location, such as the nose, lip, or cheek. Occasionally bleomycin can improve the appearance of a facial lesion by 10% to 15% and obviate the need for operative intervention.
- When resection is being considered, the postoperative scar or deformity after removal of the lymphatic malformation should not be worse than the preoperative appearance of the lesion.
- Extirpation of a lymphatic malformation can be associated with significant morbidity: major blood loss, iatrogenic injury, and deformity. For example, resection of a cervicofacial lesion can injure the facial nerve (76%) or hypoglossal nerve (24%).
- Because significant blood loss can occur during excision, local anesthetic with epinephrine is administered, and resection of an extremity lesion is performed using a tourniquet.
- A localized lymphatic malformation may be excised and the wound edges reapproximated without complex reconstruction.
- For diffuse lymphatic malformations, staged resection of defined anatomic regions is recommended. Subtotal excisions of problematic areas, such as bleeding vesicles or an overgrown lip, should be carried out rather than an attempting "complete" removal, which would result in a worse deformity than the malformation.
- Lymphatic malformations involving the head and neck may be resected using a coronal (forehead, orbit), tarsal (eyelid), preauricular-melolabial-transoral (cheek), or transverse mucosal (lip) incision.

- A radical neck approach is required for cervical lymphatic malformation to preserve important structures.
- Macroglossia may require tongue reduction to return the tongue to the oral cavity or to correct an open-bite deformity.
- Operative intervention for bone overgrowth is required in 75% of patients with a cervicofacial lymphatic malformation. Bony hypertrophy is corrected by osseous contouring. Malocclusion may necessitate orthognathic correction, usually at the time of skeletal maturity (16 years in girls, 18 years in boys).
- Most wounds are amenable to linear closure by advancing skin flaps. Skin grafts may be necessary to cover large areas (Fig. 9-4). Wounds may be allowed to heal secondarily; the increased scar might help to minimize a recurrence.
- Postoperative drainage, seroma, and infection are minimized using drains and compression garments.

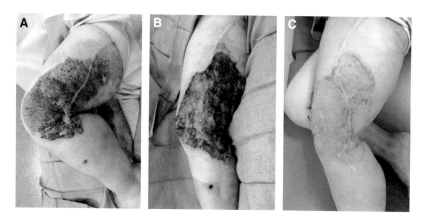

Fig. 9-4   Management of microcystic lymphatic malformation. **A,** A 7-year-old boy with a diffuse microcystic lymphatic malformation of the lower extremity causing bleeding and drainage. **B,** Intraoperative image following resection and placement of a split-thickness skin graft. **C,** The healed skin graft 6 months postoperatively.

- Bleeding or leaking vesicles may be treated by carbon dioxide laser, sclerotherapy, or resection. Large areas for which carbon dioxide laser and/or sclerotherapy treatments have failed may require wide resection and skin graft coverage. Small areas can be resected and closed by direct approximation of tissues.
- Microcystic vesicles involving the oral cavity respond well to radiofrequency ablation.
- Patients and families are counseled that lymphatic malformations can expand after any intervention, and thus additional treatments may be required.

Selected References

Arnold R, Chaudry G. Diagnostic imaging of vascular anomalies. Clin Plast Surg 38:21-29, 2011.

Burrows PE, Mitri RK, Alomari A, Padua HM, Lord DJ, Sylvia MB, Fishman SJ, Mulliken JB. Percutaneous sclerotherapy of lymphatic malformations with doxycycline. Lymphat Res Biol 6:209-216, 2008.

Choi DJ, Alomari AI, Chaudry G, Orbach DB. Neurointerventional management of low-flow vascular malformations of the head and neck. Neuroimag Clin N Am 19:199-218, 2009.

Greene AK, Perlyn C, Alomari AI. Management of lymphatic malformations. Clin Plast Surg 38:75-82, 2011.

Gupta A, Kozakewich H. Histopathology of vascular anomalies. Clin Plast Surg 38:31-44, 2011.

Kim SW, Kavanagh K, Orbach DB, Alomari AI, Mulliken JB, Rahbar R. Long-term outcome of radiofrequency ablation for intraoral microcystic lymphatic malformation. Arch Otolaryngol Head Neck Surg 137:1247-1250, 2011.

Lala S, Mulliken JB, Alomari AI, Fishman SJ, Kozakewich HP, Chaudry G. Gorham-Stout disease and generalized lymphatic anomaly—clinical, radiologic, and histologic differentiation. Skeletal Radiol (in press).

Smith MC, Zimmerman B, Burke DK, Bauman NM, Sato Y, Smith RJ. Efficacy and safety of OK-432 immunotherapy of lymphatic malformations. Laryngoscope 119:107-115, 2009.

10

Primary Lymphedema

TUMORS	MALFORMATIONS		
	Slow-Flow	Fast-Flow	Overgrowth Syndromes
Infantile Hemangioma	*Capillary Malformation*	*Arteriovenous Malformation*	CLOVES Klippel- Trenaunay Maffucci Parkes Weber Proteus Sturge-Weber
Congenital Hemangioma	***Lymphatic Malformation*** Macrocystic Microcystic Combined (macrocystic/ microcystic) ***Primary lymphedema*** Gorham-Stout disease Generalized lymphatic anomaly Kaposiform lymphangiomatosis		
Kaposiform Hemangioendothelioma	*Venous Malformation*		
Pyogenic Granuloma			
Rare Vascular Tumors			

CLINICAL FEATURES

- Primary (idiopathic) lymphedema is a type of lymphatic malformation. Malformed lymphatic vessels (usually hypoplastic) in an extremity or genitalia cause accumulation of protein-rich fluid in the interstitial space. The affected area becomes swollen and then enlarges because of progressive subcutaneous adipose deposition (Fig. 10-1).
- The condition is rare (1.2/100,000 persons less than 20 years of age). Males and females are affected equally.
- Lymphedema is painless and ulceration is rare. There is no cure.
- Secondary lymphedema is not a vascular anomaly and results from injury to lymphatic vessels or axillary/inguinal lymph nodes. The most common causes are radiation and/or lymphadenectomy for cancer treatment, and a parasitic infection.
- Primary lymphedema can present during infancy, childhood, adolescence, or adulthood (Table 10-1).

Table 10-1 *Onset of Primary Lymphedema*

HISTORIC CLASSIFICATION		CURRENT DEVELOPMENTAL CLASSIFICATION	
Age of Onset	**Definition**	**Age of Onset**	**Definition**
Congenital	At birth Birth-3 months Birth-1 year Birth-2 years	Infancy	Birth-1 year
Praecox	Birth-35 years Any time after birth After birth-24 years After birth-35 years 4 months-20 years 1 year-35 years	Childhood	1-8 years (females) 1-9 years (males)
		Adolescence	9-21 years (females) 10-21 years (males)
Tarda	After 20 years After 35 years	Adulthood	After 21 years

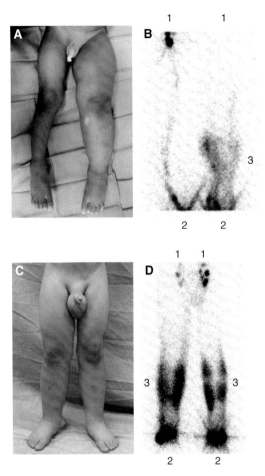

Fig. 10-1   Primary lymphedema. **A,** Male infant with left lower extremity lymphedema present at birth. **B,** His lymphoscintigram image, obtained 30 minutes after injection of radiolabeled tracer into the feet, shows normal transit to the inguinal nodes in the right lower extremity and no transport to the inguinal nodes on the left side with dermal backflow. **C,** Male child with bilateral lower extremity and scrotal lymphedema present at birth. **D,** His lymphoscintigram image, obtained 2 hours after injection, shows minimal uptake in the inguinal nodes and bilateral dermal backflow (normal transit time to the inguinal lymph nodes is 45 minutes). (*1,* Inguinal nodes; *2,* injection site into the feet; *3,* dermal backflow.)

- The terms *congenital, praecox,* and *tarda,* previously used to define age of onset, are neither standardized nor precise and thus should be abandoned.
- In the pediatric population, onset occurs in infancy (49.2%), childhood (9.5%), or adolescence (41.3%). Males are more likely to present in infancy (68%), whereas females most commonly develop the disease during adolescence (55%).
- The lower extremities are affected in 91.7% of patients (50% have unilateral disease, and 50% have bilateral lymphedema); 18% have genital lymphedema (usually associated with lower extremity disease); 4% have isolated genital involvement; and 16% have upper extremity disease. Rarely, a child can have lymphedema affecting the legs, genitalia, and arms. Bilateral lower extremity lymphedema is more common in patients presenting in infancy (63%), compared to adolescence (30%).
- 12% of patients with primary lymphedema have a familial or syndromic association, such as Turner syndrome or Milroy disease.
- Patients with a *FOXC2* mutation causing lymphedema distichiasis have an extra row of eyelashes and may exhibit eyelid ptosis and/or yellow nails.
- Hypotrichosis-lymphedema-telangiectasia (*SOX18* mutation) causes sparse hair and cutaneous telangiectasias and can have dominant or recessive transmission.
- Hennekam syndrome (*CCBE1* mutation) is characterized by generalized lymphedema with visceral involvement, developmental delay, flat face, hypertelorism, and a broad nasal bridge.
- Milroy disease denotes an infant with lower extremity lymphedema (unilateral or bilateral) present at birth with either a positive family history or a documented mutation in *VEGFR3* without a family history of the disease.
- Meige disease refers to familial lymphedema of the lower extremity that presents in adolescence. Because a mutation for this condition has not been identified, a diagnosis of Meige disease should not be used for patients with adolescent-onset lymphedema without a family history of the disease.

- Lymphedema is progressive. The distal limb is always affected and swelling can migrate proximally. Initially pitting edema is present, but over time the edema is replaced by subcutaneous adipose tissue, and the circumference of the extremity increases. Fat in an extremity can be elevated by 73%. Only tissues above the muscle fascia are affected. Twenty-five percent of children who present with unilateral lower limb lymphedema develop the condition in the contralateral extremity.
- The two major morbidities caused by lymphedema are:
  1. Psychosocial problems because the overgrown limb can cause a deformity.
  2. Infection resulting from lymph stagnation, impaired immunosurveillance, decreased oxygen delivery, and a proteinaceous environment favorable to bacterial growth.
- A lymphedematous extremity has approximately a 70 times increased risk of cellulitis compared with the nonaffected limb; 19% of patients have a history of cellulitis, 13% have been hospitalized, and 7% have more than three attacks each year.
- As the size of the affected area increases, patients can have difficulty using the extremity because of its weight. It also becomes hard to find clothes that fit adequately.
- 15% of patients have cutaneous morbidity: hyperkeratosis, lymphorrhea, bleeding from vesicles, verrucous changes.
- Only 5% of affected children have orthopedic problems, such as disturbance of gait or restriction of joint motion.
- Axial overgrowth does not occur; thus patients do not need to be monitored for a leg-length discrepancy.
- 16% of males with genital lymphedema complain of dysuria, urethritis, and/or phimosis.
- Chronic lymphedema can predispose an individual to lymphangiosarcoma in the affected extremity, although the risk is very low (approximately 0.07% to 0.45%). Stewart-Treves syndrome classically refers to a lymphangiosarcoma arising in a lymphedematous upper extremity after treatment for breast cancer. The tumor can also develop in chronic lower extremity lymphedema resulting from inguinal radiation and/or lymphadenectomy.

- Lymphangiosarcoma has been described in patients with primary lymphedema (in both the upper and lower extremity). The prognosis is poor because of pulmonary metastasis and local recurrence. Mean survival is less than 2 years following diagnosis. If metastases are not present on imaging, early amputation may allow long-term survival. Chemotherapy and radiation have minimal efficacy.

ETIOPATHOGENESIS

- Several germline mutations can cause primary lymphedema: *VEGFR3* (Milroy), *FOXC2* (lymphedema distichiasis), *SOX18* (hypotrichosis-lymphedema-telangiectasia), and *CCBE1* (Hennekam).
- *VEGFR3* mutations are typically autosomal dominant, but recessive transmission can also occur. *FOXC2* is autosomal dominant, *SOX18* can be dominant or recessive, and *CCBE1* can be dominant or recessive.
- The lymphedematous limb or genitalia enlarges over time because the high-protein fluid in the interstitial space causes inflammation, fibrosis, and progressive adipose deposition. Monocytes/macrophages are recruited to areas of lymph stasis and stimulate production of proteins regulating adipose differentiation (for example, CCAAT/enhancer-binding protein-α, adiponectin, and peroxisome proliferator–activated receptor-γ).

DIAGNOSIS

History and Physical Examination

- 90% of patients are diagnosed by history and physical examination.
- Males are more likely to present during infancy, whereas in females the disease onset is usually in adolescence.
- The distal extremity is always involved.

- Patients have a positive Stemmer sign: the inability to pinch the dorsal skin of the hand or foot because of edema and dermal thickening.
- A double row of eyelashes indicates lymphedema-distichiasis syndrome.
- The term *lymphedema* is commonly misused to describe any condition that causes overgrowth of a limb. Approximately a third of patients referred to our center with "lymphedema" have another condition.
- The differential diagnosis of lymphedema includes macrocystic/microcystic lymphatic malformation, capillary malformation with overgrowth, Klippel-Trenaunay syndrome, Parkes Weber syndrome, lipedema, hemihypertrophy, venous malformation, venous stasis, rheumatologic disorder, and trauma (such as ligament sprain) (Box 10-1).

Box 10-1 *Differential Diagnosis of Extremity Enlargement in Pediatric Patients Referred With "Lymphedema"*

Capillary malformation
Hemihypertrophy
Infantile hemangioma
Kaposiform hemangioendothelioma
Klippel-Trenaunay syndrome
Lipedema
Lipofibromatosis
Lymphatic malformation
Noneponymous combined vascular malformation (for example, lymphatic-venous malformation)
Obesity
Parkes Weber syndrome
Posttraumatic swelling (for example, ligament sprain, occult fracture)
Rheumatologic disease (for example, tenosynovitis, rheumatoid arthritis)
Systemic causes of edema (for example, cardiac, renal, hepatic disease)
Venous malformation
Venous stasis disease

Imaging

- Almost all patients who are suspected of having lymphedema undergo lymphoscintigraphy to obtain diagnostic confirmation and quantitatively assess lymphatic dysfunction.
- Lymphoscintigraphy is 100% specific and 92% sensitive for lymphedema. The test is not associated with morbidity. A radio-labeled colloid (usually Tc-99m filtered sulfur) is injected into the dorsum of the hand or foot. Because of the large size of the protein, it is only taken up by lymphatic vessels. Delayed transit time to the regional lymph nodes (more than 45 minutes), dermal backflow, and collateral lymphatic channels represent abnormal proximal lymphatic transport and lymphedema.
- Lymphangiography, the injection of dye into the lymphatic vasculature, is no longer used to evaluate lymphedema because it is technically difficult to perform, an allergic reaction to the dye can occur, lymphangitis is common (19%), and it may worsen the lymphedema (32%). A lymphangiogram may be indicated to identify a localized anatomic obstruction in the thoracic duct if a bypass procedure is planned.
- MRI and CT are neither sensitive nor specific for lymphedema. These studies are only obtained to determine the amount of subcutaneous adipose tissue present if an excisional procedure is being considered and to assess for another cause of swelling if the lymphoscintigram reveals normal findings. Lymphedema appears as thickened skin and subcutaneous tissue with adipose hypertrophy, stranding, and edema. The tissues below the muscular fascia are normal (unlike Klippel-Trenaunay syndrome, Parkes Weber syndrome, hemihypertrophy, lymphatic malformation, and venous malformation).
- Ultrasonography is nondiagnostic for lymphedema, but it can be used to rule out venous disease.

Histopathology

- Lymphedema cannot be diagnosed histopathologically because findings are nonspecific.
- Biopsy shows adipose tissue with nonspecific inflammation.

MANAGEMENT

Nonoperative Treatment

- Although there is no cure for lymphedema, most patients with primary disease are managed successfully with conservative therapy and do not require operative intervention.
- Nonoperative management includes patient education/activities of daily living and compression of the affected area.
- Patients are advised to moisturize the limb or genitalia to prevent desiccation and subsequent skin breakdown that can cause cellulitis.
- Protective clothing is worn to avoid incidental trauma that can lead to cellulitis (for example, patients with lower extremity disease should not walk barefoot).
- Exercise is encouraged, and patients are allowed to participate in all activities. Exercise improves lymphedema by stimulating muscle contraction and proximal lymph flow. Patients should maintain a normal body mass index, because obesity can worsen and cause lymphedema.
- There are no dietary restrictions, although a low-salt, low-fat diet is likely beneficial, because obesity can worsen lymphedema.
- Diuretics are ineffective and can exacerbate the disease by increasing the concentration of interstitial protein.
- Coumarin, a benzopyrone immunomodulator, is not recommended because it has minimal efficacy and may cause hepatotoxicity.
- Patients with more than three episodes of cellulitis each year may benefit from long-term suppressive antibiotic therapy against *Streptococcus*.

Compression

- The mainstay of treatment for lymphedema is compression, which decreases the size of the area by reducing edema and slows progression of the disease by minimizing the high-protein fluid in the interstitial space, which stimulates adipose deposition.
- Pressure may reduce extremity volume by increasing lymph transport, decreasing capillary filtration, opening collapsed vessels, minimizing interstitial pressure, and/or widening the vessel wall by direct injury.
- Static compression produced by custom-fitted garments is the most effective compression method, because the garments are worn continuously. When they are progressively tightened (controlled compression therapy), extremity volume may be reduced by 47% over 1 year. A single-layer garment is used for the upper extremity (30 mm Hg), and two layers are applied to the lower extremity (a 20 mm Hg garment over a 30 mm Hg sleeve). Patients with genital lymphedema are advised to wear a tight-fitting athletic undergarment.
- Pneumatic compression devices deliver intermittent pressure through a power source and an inflatable sleeve. Machines may be sequential or nonsequential, gradient or nongradient, and have single or multiple compartments. A sequential pump has multiple chambers that inflate distally, followed by the expansion of more proximal chambers. A gradient pump delivers more force in the distal chambers. We prefer a sequential, gradient device with multiple compartments, because it best recapitulates physiologic lymph flow. Extremity volume may be reduced 3% to 66% using pneumatic compression. We recommend pumping for at least 2 hours per day.
- For manual lymphatic drainage, massage is used to stimulate proximal lymphatic flow. This technique has minimal efficacy (10% reduction in limb volume) and is less likely to be effective for patients with moderate or chronic lymphedema after fibro-adipose deposition has occurred. Disadvantages of this treatment modality include its substantial time burden for patients, reliance on a provider for treatment, and cost.

- Combination compressive regimens (for example, complex decongestive therapy) are programs that combine skin care, manual lymphatic drainage, and compression bandaging. A treatment phase of several weeks at an outpatient facility is initiated, followed by a maintenance phase conducted at home by the patient or family. Limb volume may be reduced 19% to 68% but disadvantages include its substantial time burden for patients, reliance on a provider for treatment, and cost.
- We prescribe custom-fitted garments and pneumatic compression for our patients, rather than manual lymphatic drainage/combination compressive regimens, because their efficacy is superior, they are easier for the patient, and treatment is not dependent on a therapist.

Timing of Operative Intervention

- Operative intervention is rarely indicated for patients with primary lymphedema. It is more common for individuals with genital disease (36%) than for patients with extremity lymphedema (6%).
- Patients are only considered for a surgical procedure if they have been compliant with conservative therapies and have significant morbidity despite maximal conservative interventions.
- Indications for a surgical procedure include recurrent infections, enlargement of the extremity or genitalia inhibits daily activities or the ability to wear normal clothing, or the patient is unhappy with the appearance of the affected area.
- Pubertal males often seek improvement for the appearance of their genitalia, whereas adolescent females are interested in improving the contour of their extremity.
- There are two categories of operative intervention: physiologic and excisional.
- Physiologic procedures attempt to produce new lymphatic connections to enhance lymph drainage. Excisional operations remove excessive subcutaneous fibroadipose tissue with or without overlying skin.

- We prefer excisional procedures because they have consistent and excellent long-term results. In addition, all patients (minor, moderate, or severe disease) are potential candidates. Suction-assisted lipectomy (liposuction) is our preferred technique. We reserve staged skin and subcutaneous resection for patients with very severe disease.
- It is possible that excisional procedures may also have a physiologic benefit by reducing the amount of lymph load produced by the extremity, increasing drainage from the superficial to deep system by removing intervening tissue, and increasing blood flow to the skin because the procedures delay the integument.
- Physiologic procedures have poor results for moderate to severe lymphedema. In early disease, results are inconsistent, and long-term benefits are modest. Even if improved proximal lymph flow is achieved, the excess fibroadipose tissue cannot be reversed and may only be improved using an excisional operation.

Physiologic Procedures

- Physiologic procedures are done to attempt to reconnect, reconstruct, or stimulate lymphatic pathways.
- Handley (1908) unsuccessfully used subcutaneous silk threads to drain edematous areas into normal tissue.
- Kondoleon (1915) removed the muscle fascia in an attempt to allow the superficial lymphatics to drain into the deep lymphatic system. His procedure did not prove successful.
- Flap transpositions to connect superficial lymphatics to the deep system have been abandoned because clear efficacy has not been proven, and the procedures have greater morbidity compared with excisional or microsurgical operations. Examples include the Thompson procedure (1962), which buried a skin flap into muscle; the use of an omental flap to drain the axillary/inguinal lymph nodes (Goldsmith, 1967); and a myocutaneous flap transposition (rectus abdominis muscle) into the groin.

- Microsurgical lymphatic-venous anastomosis (LVA) is the most commonly performed physiologic procedure. Results are variable, but reported improvement for minor to moderate disease is 55% excess volume reduction. If LVA is performed, it should be carried out early in the disease when there is still potentially functional drainage, before progressive fibrosis and adipose deposition occur.
- Recently microsurgical lymph node transfer from the inguinal nodes to the axilla has been performed. Although beneficial results have been reported, these patients had early disease, and the contribution of postoperative manual lymphatic drainage to the improvement is unclear. Lymphoscintigraphy also failed to show improved lymphatic function in most patients. This procedure also risks causing donor site lymphedema in the lower extremity, where the nodes were harvested; lymphedema occurs in 2% of patients following sentinel node biopsy.

Excisional Procedures

- Excisional procedures are performed to remove excess fat, fibrous tissue, and expanded skin that develops with lymphedema.
- Because the underlying disease is not cured, lifelong compression therapy is required to minimize edema, inflammation, and recurrent fibroadipose deposition.
- Suction-assisted lipectomy (liposuction) is our first-line operative intervention for extremity lymphedema because of its efficacy, consistent results, and low morbidity (Fig. 10-2). Excess volume reduction for upper extremity lymphedema can be as high as 106% after 1 year, with no recurrence 15 years postoperatively. Suction-assisted lipectomy for lower extremity lymphedema achieves 75% volume reduction 18 months postoperatively. Liposuction increases cutaneous blood flow, reduces the annual risk of cellulitis by 30%, and significantly improves quality of life. Lymphatics are not injured by the procedure, and lymph flow is not affected.

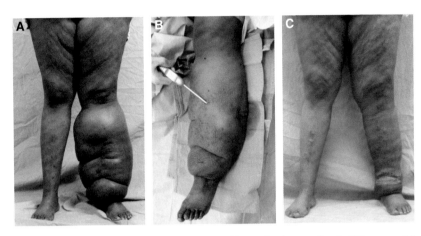

Fig. 10-2 Operative management of lymphedema. **A,** A 37-year-old woman with adolescent-onset primary lymphedema of the left lower extremity. **B,** Removal of excess subcutaneous adipose tissue using suction-assisted lipectomy. **C,** Improved contour 5 months postoperatively.

- Staged cutaneous and subcutaneous excision is used for severe extremity lymphedema with significant skin excess or for genital lymphedema. Sistrunk (1918) modified the Kondoleon procedure (excision of deep fascia) by excising extensive tissue and fascia. Homans (1936) removed subcutaneous tissue and deep fascia and created thin skin flaps. Miller (1998) showed significant improvement in limb size in 79% of patients and a reduction in the risk of infection. Postoperative lymphoscintigraphy showed increased lymphatic function, suggesting that this procedure also has physiologic benefit.

- The disadvantages of cutaneous and subcutaneous extremity resection, compared with suction-assisted lipectomy, include the following:
  - Two stages are required.
  - An extended hospital stay is necessary.
  - Incisions/scars are long.
  - There is greater operative morbidity.

Selected References

Boon LM, Ballieux F, Vikkula M. Pathogenesis of vascular anomalies. Clin Plast Surg 38:7-19, 2011.

Brorson H, Ohlin K, Olsson G, Svensson B, Svensson H. Controlled compression and liposuction treatment for lower extremity lymphedema. Lymphology 41:52-63, 2008.

Greene AK, Schook CC. Primary lymphedema: definition of onset based on developmental age. Plast Reconstr Surg 129:221e-222e, 2012.

Greene AK, Slavin SA, Borud L. Treatment of lower extremity lymphedema with suction-assisted lipectomy. Plast Reconstr Surg 118:118e-121e, 2006.

Schook CC, Mulliken JB, Fishman SJ, Alomari AI, Greene AK. Differential diagnosis of lower extremity lymphedema in 170 pediatric patients. Plast Reconstr Surg 127:1571-1581, 2011.

Schook CC, Mulliken JB, Fishman SJ, Grant F, Zurakowski D, Greene AK. Primary lymphedema: clinical features and management in 138 pediatric patients. Plast Reconstr Surg 127:2419-2431, 2011.

Sharma A, Schwartz RA. Stewart-Treves syndrome: pathogenesis and management. J Am Acad Dermatol 67:1342-1348, 2012.

CHAPTER 11

Venous Malformation

TUMORS	MALFORMATIONS		
	Slow-Flow	**Fast-Flow**	**Overgrowth Syndromes**
Infantile Hemangioma	*Capillary Malformation*	*Arteriovenous Malformation*	CLOVES Klippel- Trenaunay Maffucci Parkes Weber Proteus Sturge-Weber
Congenital Hemangioma	*Lymphatic Malformation*		
Kaposiform Hemangioendothelioma	*Venous Malformation* Blue rubber bleb nevus syndrome Cerebral cavernous malformation Cutaneomucosal venous malformation Diffuse phlebectasia of Bockenheimer Fibroadipose vascular anomaly Glomuvenous malformation Phlebectasia Sinus pericranii Verrucous venous malformation		
Pyogenic Granuloma			
Rare Vascular Tumors			

CLINICAL FEATURES

- Venous malformation (VM) results from an error in vascular morphogenesis. Veins are dilated, with thin walls and abnormal smooth muscle. Consequently lesions expand, flow stagnates, and clotting occurs.
- Although venous malformations are present at birth, they may not become evident until childhood or adolescence, when they have grown large enough to cause a visible deformity or symptoms.
- Lesions are blue, soft, and compressible. Hard, calcified phleboliths may be palpable.
- Venous malformations range from small, localized skin lesions to diffuse malformations involving multiple tissue planes and vital structures (Fig. 11-1).
- Venous malformations are sporadic and solitary in 90% of patients.
- A sporadic venous malformation is usually greater than 5 cm (56%), single (99%), and located on the head or neck (47%), extremities (40%), or trunk (13%).
- Almost all lesions involve the skin, mucosa, or subcutaneous tissue; 50% also affect deeper structures, such as muscle, bone, joints, or viscera.
- 10% of patients have multifocal, familial lesions: either glomuvenous malformation (GVM) (8%) or cutaneomucosal venous malformation (CMVM) (2%) (Fig. 11-2).
- Venous malformation (phlebectasia) may be a part of a combined malformation, particularly lymphatic, because lymphatics arise from veins embryologically.
- The primary morbidity of a venous malformation is psychosocial, because most lesions affect the skin and cause a deformity.
- The second most common complication associated with venous malformation is pain, caused by thrombosis and phlebolith formation. Stagnation within a venous malformation causes a localized intravascular coagulopathy and thrombosis. Symptoms

resolve after the phlebolith is resorbed. Patients with venous malformations are not at risk for thromboembolism, unless a large
phlebectatic vein is connected to the deep venous system.

• Head or neck venous malformations can present with mucosal
bleeding or progressive distortion, leading to airway or orbital
compromise.

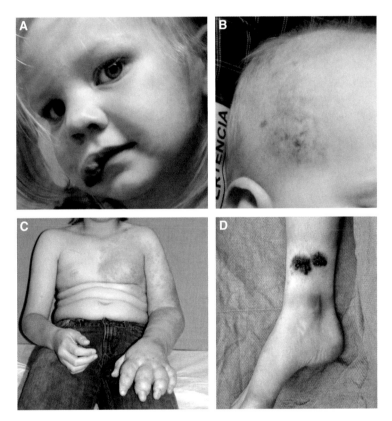

Fig. 11-1 Appearance of venous malformation. **A,** A sporadic, localized
lesion affecting the upper lip. **B,** Scalp location with sinus pericranii. **C,** Extensive venous malformation involving all structures of the upper extremity
(diffuse phlebectasia of Bockenheimer). **D,** Verrucous venous malformation
("verrucous hemangioma").

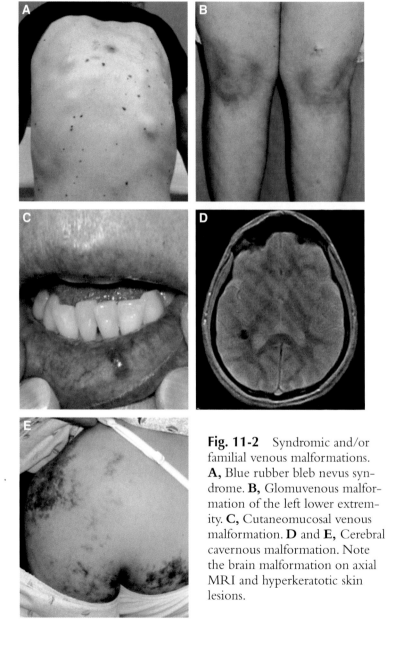

Fig. 11-2   Syndromic and/or familial venous malformations. **A,** Blue rubber bleb nevus syndrome. **B,** Glomuvenous malformation of the left lower extremity. **C,** Cutaneomucosal venous malformation. **D** and **E,** Cerebral cavernous malformation. Note the brain malformation on axial MRI and hyperkeratotic skin lesions.

- Extremity venous malformations can cause a leg-length discrepancy, hypoplasia as a result of disuse atrophy, pathologic fracture, hemarthrosis, and degenerative arthritis.
- Venous malformations involving muscle may result in fibrosis, pain, and disability.
- Gastrointestinal venous malformations can cause bleeding and chronic anemia.
- Venous malformations progress over time: 26% before adolescence, 75% prior to adulthood, and 93% during the patient's lifetime. Progression is 2.6 times more likely during adolescence (61%) than during childhood (22%). Consequently, most patients who present with asymptomatic lesions ultimately will require intervention.

ETIOPATHOGENESIS

- Venous malformations result from an error in vascular morphogenesis. Veins have decreased smooth muscle cells that are arranged in clumps rather than concentrically.
- Mutations for types of familial venous malformations are known:
  - *Glomulin* (glomuvenous malformation)
  - *TIE2* (cutaneomucosal venous malformation)
  - CCM1/*KRIT1,* CCM2/*malcavernin,* CCM3/*PDCD10* (cerebral cavernous malformation)
- 50% of sporadic venous malformations have a somatic mutation in the endothelial receptor TIE2. Angiopoietins, the ligands for *TIE2,* are involved in angiogenesis. The mutation uncouples endothelial cells and pericytes altering venous development.
- Possible causes for enlargement of a venous malformation over time include dilation of veins, angiogenesis, or vasculogenesis.
- Because lesions have a higher risk of progression during puberty, adolescent hormones might stimulate venous malformations.

PHENOTYPIC CONSIDERATIONS

Blue Rubber Bleb Nevus Syndrome (BRBNS)

- Blue rubber bleb nevus syndrome is a rare nonhereditary disease with multiple small (less than 2 cm) venous malformations involving the skin, soft tissue, and gastrointestinal tract (usually the small intestine).
- Males and females are affected equally.
- Patients can have hundreds of lesions.
- Venous malformations involve the extremities (93%), trunk (80%), or head and neck (60%).
- 80% have a dominant venous malformation involving the extremity (43%), trunk (37%), or head and neck (20%).
- 75% of patients with gastrointestinal involvement have bleeding requiring blood transfusions.
- Resection of intestinal lesions may be required.

Cerebral Cavernous Malformation (CCM)

- Cerebral cavernous malformation is a rare sporadic or inherited disorder (autosomal dominant) with venous malformations involving the brain and spinal cord.
- The condition results from a mutation in CCM1/*KRIT1*, CCM2/*malcavernin*, and/or CCM3/*PDCD10*.
- 9% of patients have skin lesions, most commonly hyperkeratotic capillary or venous malformations.
- 87% of children with skin lesions have the *KRIT1* mutation.
- These patients are at risk for development of new intracranial lesions, seizures, and hemorrhage.

Cutaneomucosal Venous Malformation (CMVM)

- Small multifocal mucocutaneous lesions caused by a gain-of-function mutation in the *TIE2* receptor.
- Autosomal dominant and less common than glomuvenous malformation.

- Lesions are small (76% are less than 5 cm), multiple (73%), and located on the head or neck (50%), extremity (37%), or trunk (13%).
- CMVMs typically affect the skin and oral mucosa but also may be located in the muscle, brain, lung, and gastrointestinal tract.
- Lesions are often asymptomatic.
- In contrast to glomuvenous malformation, the venous malformations are not as blue, are rarely hyperkeratotic, have less of a cobblestone appearance, and are not painful on palpation.

Diffuse Phlebectasia of Bockenheimer

- Diffuse phlebectasia of Bockenheimer is an extensive venous malformation affecting all tissues of an extremity—the skin, subcutaneous tissue, muscle, and bone.
- The limb is often hypoplastic.
- Hemarthropathy causing arthritis and joint destruction can occur.
- Pain may be reduced with targeted sclerotherapy to symptomatic areas.
- Joint disease is managed with arthroscopic resection and/or intraarticular sclerotherapy.
- Soft tissue resection of symptomatic areas is rarely indicated.

Fibroadipose Vascular Anomaly (FAVA)

- Fibroadipose vascular anomaly is a unique lesion that shares clinical, radiographic, and histologic features with intramuscular venous malformation.
- The condition typically affects the calf (70%), followed by the thigh (12%), forearm (8%), gluteal area (7%), and ankle or foot (3%).
- FAVA is clinically differentiated from an intramuscular venous malformation by the presence of significant pain (98%), contractures (40%), a nonspongiform venous cutaneous component (phlebectasia, capillary malformation, and/or lymphatic vesicles) (44%), and poor response to sclerotherapy.

- A fibroadipose vascular anomaly can be differentiated from an intramuscular venous malformation through these characteristics seen on MRI: the FAVA has more fat or fibrosis, is not as bright on T2 images, is more heterogeneous, has smaller, less defined channels, and displays nonspongiform-appearing vessels.
- Histopathologically, a fibroadipose vascular anomaly is more infiltrative and has greater fibroadipose tissue than a venous malformation.
- Management includes (1) aggressive physical therapy to minimize contractures; (2) corticosteroid injection into the lesion to reduce pain; and/or (3) resection.
- Sclerotherapy is not effective because a fibroadipose vascular anomaly is solid. However, if adjacent phlebectasia and thrombosis are present, sclerosing abnormal veins can alleviate pain.
- Because long-term control of symptoms is difficult to achieve with nonoperative management, most patients require resection (unlike venous malformation). During excision, neurolysis and/or neurectomy may be necessary, which can further improve neurogenic pain.

Glomuvenous Malformation (GVM)

- Glomuvenous malformation is an autosomal dominant familial condition with abnormal smooth muscle–like glomus cells along ectatic veins.
- It is caused by a loss-of-function mutation in the *glomulin* gene.
- Lesions are typically multiple (70%) and small (two thirds are less than 5 cm).
- They involve the skin and subcutaneous tissue. Approximately 50% of patients can also have intramuscular lesions.
- GVM is located on the extremities (76%), trunk (14%), or head and neck (10%).
- This condition is more painful than a typical or sporadic venous malformation (especially on palpation).
- 17% of patients develop new lesions over time.

Phlebectasia

- Phlebectasia is the abnormal dilation of a vein.
- There are three forms:
  1. Sporadic phlebectasia (congenital varicosity)
  2. Phlebectasia associated with lymphatic malformation (lymphatic-venous malformation)
  3. Syndromic phlebectasia (such as a lateral embryonal vein in Klippel-Trenaunay syndrome)
- If a phlebectatic vein communicates with the deep venous system through large perforators, thrombosis and pulmonary embolism can occur.
- Problematic phlebectatic veins are usually treated with sclerotherapy, although endovascular laser therapy and excision are other treatment options.

Sinus Pericranii

- Sinus pericranii is a venous anomaly of the scalp or face, with transcalvarial communication to the dura.
- Before resection of a soft tissue lesion, transcranial veins are obliterated endovascularly to prevent intracranial thrombosis.

Verrucous Venous Malformation (VVM)

- Verrucous venous malformation is clinically, radiographically, and histologically similar to a hyperkeratotic venous malformation.
- It is also called *verrucous hemangioma*. The term "hemangioma" has been used because some histologic features are similar to an involuted infantile hemangioma.
- Lesions range from 2 to 8 cm and affect the skin and subcutis of an extremity (91%) or trunk (9%).
- Over time it becomes more hyperkeratotic and frequently bleeds.
- The lesion is treated either by carbon dioxide laser or resection.

DIAGNOSIS

History and Physical Examination

- 90% of venous malformations are diagnosed by history and physical examination.
- The primary differential diagnosis is lymphatic malformation.
- Patients and/or family members are queried about a family history of similar lesions, especially if a glomuvenous malformation or cutaneomucosal venous malformation is suspected.
- Unlike sporadic venous malformations, familial lesions are usually smaller, multiple, and superficial. Glomuvenous malformation is painful on palpation.
- Dependent positioning of the affected area will cause a venous malformation to enlarge.
- If the diagnosis is equivocal, a handheld Doppler probe will rule out a fast-flow lesion such as a hemangioma or arteriovenous malformation.
- Small, superficial venous malformations do not require further diagnostic workup.

Imaging

- Large or deep venous malformations are evaluated by MRI to confirm the diagnosis, define the extent of the malformation, and plan treatment (Figs. 11-3 and 11-4).
- MRI sequences are obtained with fat suppression and contrast. Lesions are hypointense or isointense on T1 images and hyperintense on T2 sequences. Phleboliths demonstrate a low-intensity signal on both T1 and T2 images. Contrast helps delineate a venous malformation from a lymphatic malformation, because venous lesions enhance uniformly following gadolinium administration. Venous malformations can appear less intense after treatment because of scar tissue. Morphologically, venous malformation is often circumscribed, lobulated, and isolated to an anatomic structure (usually muscle). In contrast, a lymphatic malformation is more likely to infiltrate through several tissue planes.

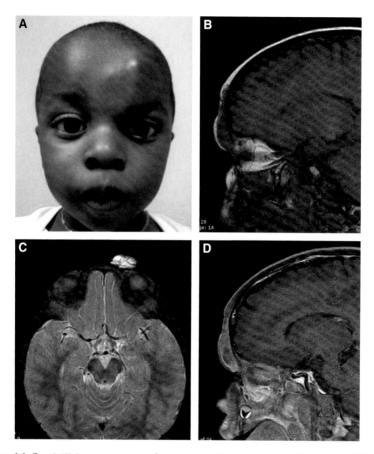

Fig. 11-3   MRI appearance of venous malformation. **A,** A 2-year-old boy with a venous malformation of the forehead. **B,** Sagittal T1 image. **C,** Axial T2 sequence shows a lobulated, hyperintense lesion. **D,** Postcontrast sagittal T1 image shows enhancement of the venous malformation.

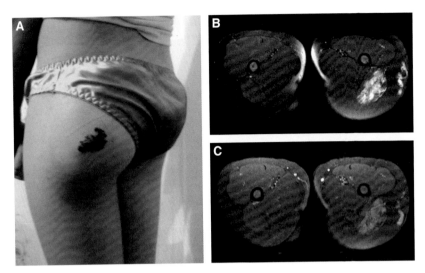

Fig. 11-4   A fibroadipose vascular anomaly. **A,** An adolescent girl with severe pain of the left buttock. Note the cutaneous malformation. **B,** T2 MR sequence shows a hyperintense lesion of the gluteus maximus muscle. **C,** T1 MR image after injection of a contrast medium shows heterogeneous enhancement. Unlike a typical intramuscular venous malformation, note the nonspongiform vessels and an associated subcutaneous lesion.

- MR venography is occasionally indicated to show the deep venous system in lesions affecting an extremity.
- Ultrasonography can be used instead of MRI for imaging of some localized venous malformations and does not require sedation in young children. Findings include compressible, anechoic-hypoechoic spaces with septations, minimal flow on color Doppler, areas separated by more solid regions of variable echogenicity, and phleboliths causing hyperechoic areas with acoustic shadowing.
- Phlebectasia is initially imaged with ultrasound to demonstrate the dilated, incompetent veins and large perforators.
- Computed tomography is occasionally indicated to assess an osseous venous malformation.

- Intralesional venography is not needed to confirm the diagnosis of a venous malformation. It is performed during sclerotherapy before sclerosant is injected.

Histopathology

- Histopathologic diagnosis of venous malformation is rarely necessary. A biopsy is indicated only if the history, physical examination, and imaging are equivocal.
- Veins are irregular and lined by flat endothelium, with a paucity of smooth muscle cells. Thrombi are commonly found in vessel lumens, and papillary endothelial hyperplasia may be present. Organized thrombi can become incorporated into the venous wall as a fibromyxoid nodule.
- A glomuvenous malformation has ectatic veins with smooth muscle replaced by single or multiple layers of cuboidal "glomus" cells.

MANAGEMENT

Nonoperative Treatment

- The natural history of venous malformation is explained to patients and families, including the possibility of expansion and phlebothrombosis.
- Patients with glomuvenous malformation or cutaneomucosal venous malformation and their family members are counseled about the risk of developing new lesions and transmitting the condition to their offspring.
- Because venous malformation is at greatest risk for expansion during adolescence, pubertal hormones may be involved in its pathogenesis. Consequently, women are advised to avoid estrogen-containing oral contraceptives, because estrogen has more potent proangiogenic activity than progesterone.
- Patients with a large extremity venous malformation are prescribed custom-fitted compression garments to reduce stagnation of blood, phlebolith formation, and pain.

- Individuals with recurrent discomfort are given low-dose (81 mg) prophylactic daily aspirin to prevent phlebothrombosis.
- Children with an extensive venous malformation are evaluated by a hematologist. Large lesions are at risk for coagulation of stagnant blood, stimulation of thrombin, and conversion of fibrinogen to fibrin. Fibrinolysis results in localized intravascular coagulopathy. Plasma D-dimers and fibrin split products are elevated. Fibrinogen, factor V, factor VIII, factor XIII, and antithrombin levels are low. Prothrombin time and activated partial thromboplastin time are normal. The chronic consumptive coagulopathy can cause either thrombosis (phleboliths) or bleeding (hemarthrosis, hematoma, or intraoperative blood loss).
- Significant bleeding or life-threatening thrombosis is rare. Almost all venous malformations are not at risk for thromboemboli, because they do not affect the deep venous system, and thrombosed lesions are sequestered from larger veins.
- Patients with extensive venous anomalies involving the deep venous system or phlebectasia, however, are at risk for thromboemboli.
- Low-molecular-weight heparin is considered for patients with significant localized intravascular coagulopathy or who are at risk for disseminated intravascular coagulation. Individuals who develop a serious thrombotic event require long-term anticoagulation therapy. An inferior or superior vena caval filter is considered for patients with contraindications to anticoagulation or who have thromboembolic events despite anticoagulation.

Timing of Intervention

- Venous malformation is a benign condition, and nonproblematic lesions can be observed.
- Intervention for a venous malformation is reserved for symptomatic lesions that cause pain, deformity, or threaten vital structures, or for asymptomatic phlebectatic areas at risk for thromboembolism.

- Many children do not require treatment at the time of diagnosis. Because venous malformations can slowly expand, patients may become symptomatic and seek intervention during late childhood or adolescence.
- Occasionally, a venous malformation involving an anatomically sensitive area or causing a significant deformity necessitates management as early as infancy. If possible, intervention should be postponed until after 12 months of age, when the risks associated with anesthesia are lower.
- Therapy for lesions causing a visible deformity should be considered before 4 years of age to limit psychological morbidity. At this time long-term memory and self-esteem begin to form.
- Some parents elect to wait until the child is older and able to make the decision to proceed with operative intervention, especially if the deformity is minor. However, if the venous malformation enlarges over time, it can become more difficult to treat.

Sclerotherapy

- Sclerotherapy involves the injection of a sclerosant into the venous malformation, which causes cellular destruction, thrombosis, and intense inflammation. Scarring leads to shrinkage of the lesion.
- The first-line treatment for a problematic venous malformation is sclerotherapy, which generally is safer and more effective than resection. Exceptions to this rule include the following:
  - Small, well-localized lesions that can be easily excised for cure
  - Glomuvenous malformations which respond less-favorably to sclerotherapy
  - Venous malformations involving the palmar aspect of the hand or adjacent to an important nerve, such as the facial nerve
- Venous malformations involving the palmar surface of the hand are best treated surgically, because if sclerotherapy is performed first, fibrosis may prohibit later operative intervention and would increase the difficulty and risks of the procedure. Similarly, if a patient requires a facial nerve dissection, previous sclerotherapy in the area of the nerve would increase the probability of nerve injury.

- Sclerotherapy provides good to excellent results in 75% to 90% of patients, reducing the size of the malformation and/or alleviating symptoms.
- Sclerotherapy is continued until symptoms are resolved and/or spaces are no longer available to inject, because the venous malformation has become fibrotic.
- Often multiple treatments are required, spaced 6 weeks apart.
- Ultrasonography is used to assess the response to treatment and to determine whether residual spaces are amenable to further injections.
- Diffuse venous malformations (Bockenheimer-type) are managed by targeting specific symptomatic areas, because the entire lesion is too extensive to treat at one time.
- Possible sclerosants include sodium tetradecyl sulfate, ethanol, polidocanol, alcohol solution of zein, bleomycin, sodium morrhuate, or ethanolamine oleate.
- We prefer sodium tetradecyl sulfate (10 ml of 3% solution mixed with 2 ml of ethiodized oil [Ethiodol] and 10 cc of air). The solution is then forced back and forth between two syringes attached to a three-way stopcock to create a foaming mixture, which increases the efficacy of the solution.
- Ethanol may be more destructive to a venous malformation than sodium tetradecyl sulfate, but it has to be carefully used because of its potential for causing local and systemic complications. The dose should not exceed 0.5 to 1 ml/kg (maximum of 30 to 60 ml). Because ethanol can cause nerve damage, it should be used with caution when injected adjacent to important structures such as the facial nerve.
- Most patients, especially children, are managed under general anesthesia with ultrasound and/or fluoroscopic guidance. A Foley catheter is placed to monitor urine output if a large venous malformation is treated. The malformation is cannulated using ultrasound, and contrast is injected under fluoroscopy to determine the anatomy of the lesion. Typically, a contrast agent (Ethiodol)

or air/carbon dioxide is mixed with the sclerosant to allow fluoroscopic or sonographic monitoring. Multiple injections into different portions of the venous malformation are often needed. Except for high-risk individuals, most patients are discharged home the day of the procedure.

- If a venous malformation has large and/or rapid drainage to adjacent veins, its outflow is occluded with external pressure or a tourniquet. Preventing the rapid distribution of the sclerosant into the systemic circulation improves the efficacy of the injection and minimizes systemic complications. Rarely, operative occlusion with sutures, platinum coils, or a liquid polymer is required to close large venous outflow channels before sclerotherapy is performed to protect important areas such as the ophthalmic veins or sinus pericranii.

- For extremity lesions, a venogram is performed to confirm the patency of the deep venous system.

- Small lesions in adolescents and adults may be treated in the office without image guidance. A 3% solution of sodium tetradecyl sulfate is diluted with saline to inject a 1% solution.

- The early response to sclerotherapy is swelling, irritation of the overlying skin, and bruising.

- The most common complication is ulceration (in less than 5% of cases), which is more likely to occur if the venous malformation involves the skin or if ethanol is used. Ulcerations are managed with local wound care and are allowed to heal secondarily. Extravasation of the sclerosant outside the lesion can cause injury to adjacent structures.

- Posttreatment swelling may necessitate close monitoring. Patients with airway lesions are admitted to the intensive care unit, and occasionally prolonged intubation or tracheostomy is required. Orbital injections can cause orbital compartment syndrome, and patients are examined by an ophthalmologist before and after the procedure. Treatment of deep extremity lesions below the muscle fascia can cause compartment syndrome.

- Systemic adverse events from sclerotherapy can occur if a significant volume of sclerosant is used: hemolysis, hemoglobinuria, and oliguria. Ethanol can cause central nervous system depression, pulmonary hypertension, hemolysis, thromboembolism, and arrhythmias.
- To prevent renal injury, D5W with 75 mEq/L of sodium bicarbonate is used to alkalinize the urine. Maintenance fluid is doubled for the first 4 hours after treatment. Oliguria is treated with one small dose of a diuretic.
- Patients with low fibrinogen levels who are at risk for thromboembolism may be given low-molecular-weight heparin (0.5 mg/kg/dose every 12 hours) for 14 days before and after the procedure (maximum 30 mg).
- Venous malformations usually reexpand after sclerotherapy; thus patients often require additional interventions over the course of their lifetime. For example, 6 months after treatment with sodium tetradecyl sulfate, 45% of patients have partial recanalization.
- Although sclerotherapy effectively reduces the size of the venous malformation and improves symptoms, it does not remove the malformation. Consequently, patients can continue to have a mass or visible deformity after treatment that may be improved by resection.

Operative Treatment

- Extirpation of a venous malformation can be associated with significant morbidity, such as major blood loss, iatrogenic injury, and deformity.
- Resection is less favorable than sclerotherapy because:
  - The entire lesion can rarely be removed.
  - Excision may cause a worse deformity than the malformation.
  - Recurrence is likely, since abnormal channels adjacent to the lesion are not treated.
  - The risk of blood loss and iatrogenic injury is high.

- Resection should be considered for:
  - Small, well-localized venous malformations that can be completely removed
  - Persistent symptoms after completion of sclerotherapy (patent channels are not accessible for further injection)
  - Lesions involving the palmar aspect of the hand or near an important nerve, such as the facial nerve, where scarring from sclerotherapy would increase the risks of later operative intervention
- When resection is being considered, the postoperative scar or deformity from removal of the venous malformation should be weighed against the preoperative appearance of the lesion.
- Almost all venous malformations should have sclerotherapy several months before operative intervention to facilitate the resection, improve the outcome, and lower the recurrence rate. Following sclerotherapy the venous malformation is replaced by scar tissue, and thus the risk of blood loss, iatrogenic injury, and recurrence is reduced. In addition, fibrosis facilitates resection and reconstruction (Fig. 11-5).
- Small, well-localized venous malformations may be removed without preoperative sclerotherapy. Because glomuvenous malformations are usually small and less amenable to sclerotherapy, the first-line therapy for symptomatic lesions often is resection.
- If a patient is receiving anticoagulation therapy, it is withheld for 12 hours before and after the intervention to prevent bleeding complications.
- When a large venous malformation is being resected, fibrinogen levels are obtained on the day of the procedure. If fibrinogen is low, cryoprecipitate may be administered.
- Verrucous venous malformation is not amenable to sclerotherapy, and thus the only treatment options are carbon dioxide laser or resection. Because lesions are often large and located on the lower extremity, serial excision or reconstruction with a skin graft may be required.

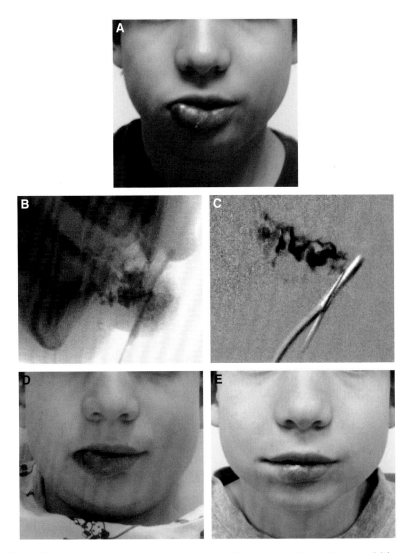

Fig. 11-5   Management of a venous malformation. **A,** A 5-year-old boy with a venous malformation of the lower lip. **B** and **C,** Contrast injection of the lesion during sclerotherapy. **D,** Improved lip contour after three sclerotherapy treatments. Further sclerotherapy was not possible, because accessible vascular channels had been obliterated. **E,** Six weeks after excision of residual fibrotic venous malformation using a transverse mucosal incision.

- Nd:YAG photocoagulation may be performed as an adjuvant to sclerotherapy for the management of difficult airway lesions.
- Gastrointestinal venous malformations with chronic bleeding, anemia, and the need for transfusion are typically managed by resection. Solitary lesions can be treated by endoscopic banding or sclerotherapy. Multifocal venous malformations, such as blue rubber bleb nevus syndrome, require removal of as many lesions as possible through multiple enterotomies, instead of bowel resection, to preserve intestinal length. Ninety percent of patients do not have recurrent bleeding after resection of individual venous malformations of the bowel. A diffuse, problematic colorectal venous malformation may require colectomy, anorectal mucosectomy, and an endorectal pull-through.
- Head and neck venous malformations are removed through the following approaches: coronal (forehead, orbit), tarsal (eyelid), preauricular-melolabial-transoral (cheek), or transverse mucosal (lip) incision.
- Because significant blood loss can occur during extirpation, local anesthetic with epinephrine should be administered, and resection of an extremity lesion is performed using a tourniquet.
- A localized venous malformation may be excised and the wound edges reapproximated without complex reconstruction. For diffuse malformations, staged resection of defined regions is recommended.
- Subtotal resections of problematic areas, such as bleeding lesions or an overgrown lip, should be carried out rather than attempting "complete" excision of a benign lesion, which would result in a worse deformity than the malformation.
- Patients and families are counseled that venous malformations can expand following excision, and thus additional operative intervention may be required.

Selected References

Adams DM. Special considerations in vascular anomalies: hematologic management. Clin Plast Surg 38:153-160, 2011.

Arnold R, Chaudry G. Diagnostic imaging of vascular anomalies. Clin Plast Surg 38:21-29, 2011.

Boon LM, Ballieux F, Vikkula M. Pathogenesis of vascular anomalies. Clin Plast Surg 38:7-19, 2011.

Boon LM, Mulliken JB, Enjolras O, Vikkula M. Glomuvenous malformation (glomangioma) and venous malformation: distinct clinicopathologic and genetic entities. Arch Dermatol 140:971-976, 2004.

Choi DJ, Alomari AI, Chaudry G, Orbach DB. Neurointerventional management of low-flow vascular malformations of the head and neck. Neuroimag Clin N Am 19:199-218, 2009.

Fishman SJ, Smithers CJ, Folkman J, Lund DP, Burrows PE, Mulliken JB, Fox VL. Blue rubber bleb nevus syndrome: surgical eradication of gastrointestinal bleeding. Ann Surg 241:523-528, 2005.

Greene AK, Alomari AI. Management of venous malformations. Clin Plast Surg 38:83-93, 2011.

Gupta A, Kozakewich H. Histopathology of vascular anomalies. Clin Plast Surg 38:31-44, 2011.

Kubiena HF, Liang MG, Mulliken JB. Genuine diffuse phlebectasia of Bockenheimer: dissection of an eponym. Pediatr Derm 23:294-297, 2006.

Limaye N, Wouters V, Uebelhoer M, Tuominen M, Wirkkala R, Mulliken JB, Eklund L, Boon LM, Vikkula M. Somatic mutations in angiopoietin receptor gene TEK cause solitary and multiple sporadic venous malformations. Nat Gen 41:118-124, 2009.

Tennant LB, Mulliken JB, Perez-Atayde AR, Kozakewich HP. Verrucous hemangioma revisited. Pediatr Dermatol 23:208-215, 2006.

Vikkula M, Boon LM, Carraway KL, Calvert JT, Diamonti AJ, Goumnerov B, Pasyk KA, Marchuk DA, Warman ML, Cantley LC, Mulliken JB, Olsen BR. Vascular dysmorphogenesis caused by an activating mutation in the receptor tyrosine kinase TIE2. Cell 87:1181-1190, 1996.

CHAPTER 12

Arteriovenous Malformation

TUMORS	MALFORMATIONS		
	Slow-Flow	**Fast-Flow**	**Overgrowth Syndromes**
Infantile Hemangioma	*Capillary Malformation*	***Arteriovenous Malformation*** Capillary malformation–arteriovenous malformation Hereditary hemorrhagic telangiectasia *PTEN*-associated vascular anomaly Wyburn-Mason syndrome	CLOVES Klippel-Trenaunay Maffucci Parkes Weber Proteus Sturge-Weber
Congenital Hemangioma	*Lymphatic Malformation*		
Kaposiform Hemangioendothelioma	*Venous Malformation*		
Pyogenic Granuloma			
Rare Vascular Tumors			

CLINICAL FEATURES

- An arteriovenous malformation (AVM) results from an error in vascular development during embryogenesis. An absent capillary bed causes shunting of blood directly from the arterial to venous circulation through a fistula (direct connection of an artery to a vein) or nidus (abnormal channels bridging the feeding artery to the draining veins) (Fig. 12-1).
- The most common site of extracranial arteriovenous malformation is the head and neck, followed by the limbs, trunk, and viscera.
- Although present at birth, an arteriovenous malformation may not become evident until childhood, after it has enlarged or become symptomatic.
- Lesions have a pink-red cutaneous stain, are warm, have a palpable thrill or bruit, and may initially be mistaken for a hemangioma or capillary malformation.
- Arteriovenous shunting reduces capillary oxygen delivery, causing ischemia. Patients are at risk for pain, ulceration, bleeding, and congestive heart failure.
- Arteriovenous malformations can cause disfigurement, destruction of tissues, and obstruction of vital structures.
- Bleeding most commonly occurs at the skin or mucosal surfaces from erosion into a superficial component of the lesion.
- High-pressure shunting of blood can cause venous hemorrhage. Arteries may rupture in weakened areas, such as aneurysms.

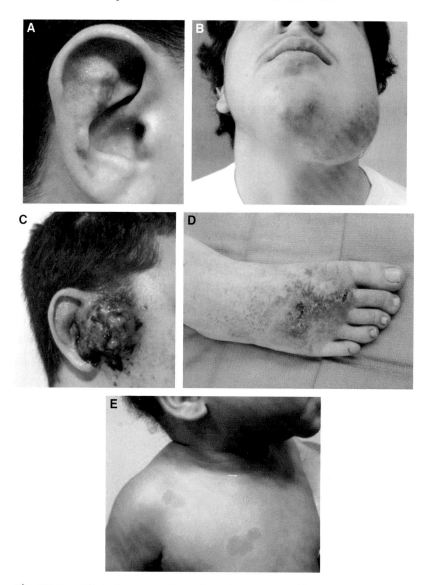

Fig. 12-1   Clinical presentation of arteriovenous malformation. **A,** Stage I lesion of the ear. **B,** Stage II enlarging submandibular arteriovenous malformation. **C,** Stage III ulcerated, painful, bleeding lesion. **D,** Stage III painful arteriovenous malformation of the foot. **E,** This infant has a capillary malformation–arteriovenous malformation (CM-AVM). Note the cutaneous stains with surrounding halos.

Table 12-1	*Schobinger Staging of Arteriovenous Malformations*
STAGE	**CLINICAL FINDINGS**
I (quiescence)	Warm, pink-blue, shunting on Doppler
II (expansion)	Enlargement, pulsation, tortuous veins
III (destruction)	Ulceration, bleeding, pain
IV (decompensation)	Cardiac failure

Adapted from Mulliken JB, Fishman SJ, Burrows PE. Vascular anomalies. Curr Prob Surg 37:517-584, 2000.

- Arteriovenous malformations progress over time and are classified according to the Schobinger staging system (Table 12-1).
- Trauma, embolization, and resection can cause an arteriovenous malformation to enlarge because of ischemia.

ETIOPATHOGENESIS

- An arteriovenous malformation may result from an error of vascular development between the fourth and sixth weeks of gestation.
- Arteriovenous channels in the primitive retiform plexus might fail to regress. This hypothesis is supported by the observation that arteriovenous malformations are 20 times more common in the central nervous system, where apoptosis is rare.
- Causative mutations for certain types of familial arteriovenous malformations have been found. Hereditary hemorrhagic telan-

giectasia results from mutations in *ENG, ACVRL1/ALK1,* and *SMAD4* that affect transforming growth factor-beta signaling. Capillary malformation–arteriovenous malformation is caused by a mutation in *RASA1. PTEN*-associated vascular anomaly results from a mutation in *PTEN.*

- Theories to explain the mechanism by which arteriovenous malformation progresses over time and recurs after treatment include:
  - Collateralization and dilation/thickening of vessels because of shunting of blood
  - Opening of latent arteriovenous shunts
  - Aneurysm formation in arteries and veins
  - Growth of new blood vessels from preexisting vasculature (angiogenesis)
  - De novo formation of new vasculature (vasculogenesis)
- Recent evidence supports the theory that vasculogenesis may be involved in the enlargement of arteriovenous malformations. Higher-staged lesions contain endothelial progenitor cells and have greater expression of vasculogenic factors, compared with lower-staged lesions. Hypoxia in the nidus may cause recruitment of endothelial progenitor cells, because ischemia is a potent stimulator of vasculogenesis. This hypothesis is supported by the observation that an arteriovenous malformation will enlarge after ischemia from proximal arterial ligation or trauma.
- Because both males and females have a twofold risk of progression in adolescence, increased circulating hormones during this period might promote the expansion of an arteriovenous malformation. This is supported by the observation that arteriovenous malformations have elevated expression of growth hormone receptors on their endothelium.

PHENOTYPIC CONSIDERATIONS

Capillary Malformation–Arteriovenous Malformation (CM-AVM)

- An autosomal dominant familial condition that affects 1/100,000 individuals.
- Patients have atypical capillary malformations that are small, multifocal, round, and pinkish-red; 50% are surrounded by a pale halo. A handheld Doppler probe usually reveals fast-flow in the lesions.
- The condition is caused by a loss-of-function mutation in *RASA1*. This gene encodes p120 RasGAP, which inhibits RAS p21 control of cellular proliferation, survival, and differentiation. Not all patients with clinically evident CM-AVM will show a *RASA1* mutation, suggesting that unknown mutations in *RASA1* or other genes may result in the same phenotype.
- An individual may have as many as 53 capillary malformations, ranging in size from 1 to 15 cm; 6% of patients have only one lesion.
- 30% of children also have an arteriovenous malformation: Parkes Weber syndrome (12%), extracerebral arteriovenous malformation (11%), or intracerebral arteriovenous malformation (7%).
- 80% of the arteriovenous malformations involve the head and neck. Patients may also have spinal arteriovenous lesions. Radiographically and histopathologically, arteriovenous malformations are similar to nonfamilial lesions. Although the capillary malformations are rarely problematic, associated arteriovenous malformations can cause significant morbidity.
- Parkes Weber syndrome consists of a diffuse extremity arteriovenous malformation that causes overgrowth of the limb. One lower extremity is usually affected, and a capillary malformation is present over the arteriovenous malformation.

- Intracranial arteriovenous malformations are associated with vein of Galen aneurysmal malformations, seizures, hydrocephalus, and developmental delay.
- Capillary malformation–arteriovenous malformation has a high penetrance (98%), although phenotypic heterogeneity is common within families (for instance, one individual may have many capillary malformations, whereas another has only Parkes Weber syndrome).
- 5% of patients with capillary malformation–arteriovenous malformation have a tumor that usually involves the nervous system (neurofibroma, optic glioma, vestibular schwannoma).
- Diagnosis of capillary malformation–arteriovenous malformation is made by history and physical examination. Patients have multifocal capillary malformations, with or without a family history of similar lesions. The capillary malformations are small, round, and usually surrounded by a halo. Doppler examination shows fast-flow, which is not present in sporadic capillary malformations.
- A patient suspected of having capillary malformation–arteriovenous malformation should undergo physical examination for arteriovenous malformations.
- Because patients with capillary malformation–arteriovenous malformation are at risk for intracranial and spinal fast-flow lesions, an MRI of the brain and spine is performed.
- Exploratory imaging of other anatomical areas is unnecessary because extracranial arteriovenous malformations do not involve the viscera.

Cobb Syndrome

- The designation *Cobb syndrome* was previously used to denote a midline capillary malformation of the posterior trunk with an underlying spinal arteriovenous malformation.
- Patients labeled with "Cobb syndrome" likely have either CLOVES syndrome or capillary malformation–arteriovenous malformation (CM-AVM).

- 28% of patients with CLOVES syndrome have spinal or paraspinal arteriovenous malformations, and truncal capillary malformations are common in this condition.
- *RASA1* mutations have been documented in patients with spinal arteriovenous malformations and overlying capillary malformations (capillary malformation–arteriovenous malformation).

Hereditary Hemorrhagic Telangiectasia (HHT)

- Hereditary hemorrhagic telangiectasia is also called *Osler-Weber-Rendu syndrome.*
- The condition is autosomal dominant and affects 1/10,000 persons.
- Mutations in endoglin *(ENG)* and activin A receptor type II–like 1 *(ACVRL1/ALK1)* cause 85% of cases. These genes are involved in transforming growth factor-beta (TGFβ) signaling.
- A mutation in *SMAD4* causes 2% of cases and is associated with juvenile polyposis (HHT/JP syndrome). *SMAD4* affects an intracellular signaling molecule in the TGFβ-bone morphogenetic protein (BMP) pathway. The causative mutations for HHT reduce smooth muscle cell recruitment to developing vessels.
- The proportion of *ENG* and *ACVRL1* mutations is equivalent. Pulmonary and cerebral arteriovenous malformations are more likely with *ENG* mutations (HHT1). Hepatic lesions are more common in patients who have *ACVRL1* mutations (HHT2). Pulmonary hypertension without significant shunting can occur in individuals with an *ACVRL1* mutation.
- Clinical findings of HHT consist of:
  – Epistaxis
  – Mucocutaneous telangiectasias (lips, oral cavity, fingers, nose)
  – Visceral arteriovenous malformations (pulmonary, cerebral, hepatic, gastrointestinal)
  – A first-degree relative with HHT
- A clinical diagnosis of HHT is considered definite if three or more findings are present, possible when a patient has two criteria, and unlikely if only one finding is present.

- Morbidity of HHT includes:
  - Upper gastrointestinal bleeding (25%)
  - Stroke and brain abscesses from pulmonary arteriovenous shunting of bacteria, air, or thrombus (the risk is greater if a feeding artery is 3 mm or larger)
  - Hemorrhage from a cerebral arteriovenous malformation (10%)
  - High-output heart failure or portal hypertension from a hepatic arteriovenous malformation (75% of patients have a liver lesion, but only 8% are symptomatic)
  - Chronic anemia, typically from epistaxis, necessitating iron supplementation and occasionally blood transfusions
- Patients with suspected HHT undergo:
  - Genetic testing to obtain a definitive diagnosis
  - Contrast echocardiography to determine the presence of pulmonary arteriovenous malformations (if present, high-resolution chest CT defines the size of the lesion; if negative, a screening chest CT is obtained every 5 years)
  - Brain MRI to rule out intracranial lesions within the first 6 months of life (if findings are negative, further screening is unnecessary)
  - Abdominal ultrasonography or CT for hepatic arteriovenous malformation, only if the patient is symptomatic
  - Endoscopy to document whether polyps are present in patients with a *SMAD4* mutation
- Management of HHT:
  - If a pulmonary arteriovenous malformation is present with a feeding artery larger than 3 mm, embolization is performed (even in asymptomatic patients) to reduce the risk of hypoxia, hemorrhage, stroke, and brain abscess.
  - If pulmonary shunting is present, prophylactic antibiotic therapy is necessary for dental cleanings and other procedures at risk for bacteremia.
  - Iron supplementation is given if a patient is anemic.
  - Problematic epistaxis is treated with laser ablation.

- Symptomatic gastrointestinal bleeding is managed by endoscopic cautery and, if that is unsuccessful, bowel resection is performed.
- Arteriovenous malformations of the brain that are larger than 1 mm are typically treated by embolization, resection, or radiation to reduce the risk of hemorrhage.
- Significant liver shunting causing high-output failure and/or hepatocyte dysfunction is treated pharmacologically (a liver transplant is indicated if medical management fails).

PTEN-Associated Vascular Anomaly (*PTEN*-AVA)

- The *PTEN* (phosphatase and tensin homolog) gene encodes a tumor suppressor lipid phosphatase involved in the phosphoinositide-3 kinase pathway that mediates cell-cycle arrest and apoptosis.
- Patients with *PTEN* mutations have *PTEN* hamartoma–tumor syndrome. The autosomal dominant condition was previously called *Cowden* or *Bannayan-Riley-Ruvalcaba syndrome*.
- Males and females are affected equally.
- 54% have a unique fast-flow vascular anomaly with arteriovenous shunting, called a *PTEN*-associated vascular anomaly (*PTEN*-AVA) (Fig. 12-2).
- Patients may have multiple *PTEN*-AVAs (57%), and 85% are intramuscular.
- Suspicion of a *PTEN*-AVA is usually prompted after reviewing the MRI or angiogram of a patient thought to have a sporadic arteriovenous malformation. Unlike a typical arteriovenous malformation, *PTEN*-AVAs can be multifocal, contain ectopic adipose tissue, and have disproportionate, segmental dilation of draining veins. Intramuscular lesions replace the architecture with disorganized fat, in contrast to nonsyndromic muscular arteriovenous malformations, which cause symmetrical overgrowth without adipose tissue.

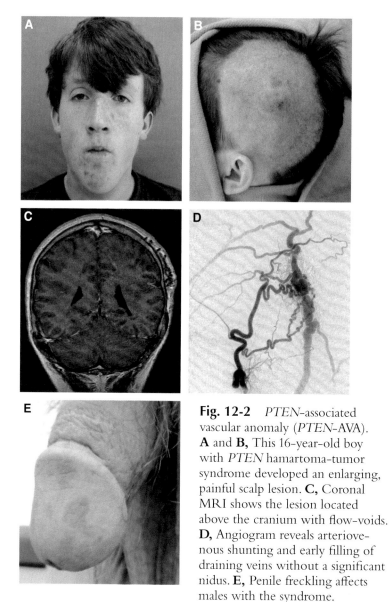

Fig. 12-2 *PTEN*-associated vascular anomaly (*PTEN*-AVA). **A** and **B,** This 16-year-old boy with *PTEN* hamartoma–tumor syndrome developed an enlarging, painful scalp lesion. **C,** Coronal MRI shows the lesion located above the cranium with flow-voids. **D,** Angiogram reveals arteriovenous shunting and early filling of draining veins without a significant nidus. **E,** Penile freckling affects males with the syndrome.

- If a patient is suspected of having a *PTEN*-AVA, a physical examination is performed to determine whether he or she has *PTEN* hamartoma syndrome. Patients with this syndrome exhibit macrocephaly (above the 97th percentile), and males have penile freckling.
- Individuals are at risk for developmental delay or autism (19%), thyroid lesions (31%), and gastrointestinal polyps (30%).
- If findings on physical examination are consistent with *PTEN* hamartoma syndrome, molecular testing is performed because patients are at risk for developing neoplasms and surveillance is required. Genetic testing is confirmative, although a germline mutation is not found in 9% of patients clinically diagnosed with *PTEN* hamartoma–tumor syndrome. Families are counseled about the risk of transmitting the mutation to their offspring.
- Patients with a *PTEN* mutation are followed closely for the presence of tumors, particularly endocrine and gastrointestinal malignancies. Endocrinology and gastroenterology consultations are obtained.
- Biopsy may aid the diagnosis of a *PTEN*-AVA. Histopathology shows skeletal muscle infiltration with adipose tissue, fibrous bands, and lymphoid aggregates. Tortuous arteries with transmural muscular hyperplasia and clusters of abnormal veins with variable smooth muscle are present.
- Symptomatic *PTEN*-AVAs are managed similarly to nonsyndromic arteriovenous malformations (embolization and/or resection). The recurrence rate after intervention is even higher than for nonsyndromic arteriovenous malformations, possibly because the loss of the tumor suppressor protein favors cellular proliferation in the lesion.

Wyburn–Mason Syndrome

- Wyburn–Mason syndrome consists of retinal arteriovenous malformations with or without a brain arteriovenous malformation or a facial vascular malformation (capillary malformation or arteriovenous malformation) (Fig. 12-3).

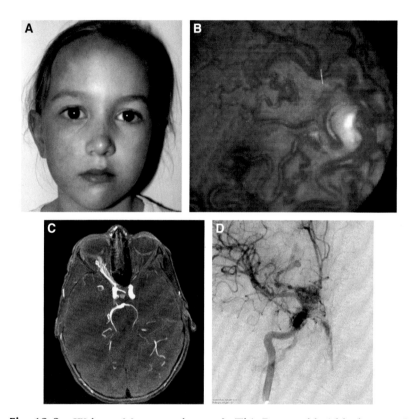

Fig. 12-3 Wyburn–Mason syndrome. **A,** This 7-year-old girl had a stage I arteriovenous malformation of the right side of the face since birth, as well as arteriovenous malformations of the retina, optic tract, and midbrain. **B,** An image of the retina shows dilated, tortuous arterioles and veins. **C,** MRI of the arteriovenous malformation extending from the globe to the brain. **D,** Angiogram shows the nidus of the arteriovenous malformation.

- Also called *Bonnet-Dechaume-Blanc syndrome* or *retinocephalofacial vascular malformation syndrome.*
- The condition is rare (approximately 121 cases in the literature), sporadic, and has an equal sex distribution.
- 22% of patients have "typical" findings of the disease: arteriovenous malformations of the retina and brain, as well as a vascular malformation of the face.
- 31% of affected children do not have a cutaneous lesion but exhibit arteriovenous malformations of the retina and have neurologic symptoms, with or without brain arteriovenous malformations.
- 47% of patients have retinal arteriovenous malformations without cutaneous or brain lesions.

DIAGNOSIS

History and Physical Examination

- 90% of arteriovenous malformations are diagnosed by history and physical examination.
- The primary differential diagnosis is hemangioma and capillary malformation. Unlike hemangioma, arteriovenous malformation expands after infancy. In contrast to capillary malformation, arteriovenous malformation has fast-flow.
- Handheld Doppler examination exhibits audible fast-flow and excludes slow-flow vascular malformations (such as capillary malformation, lymphatic malformation, venous malformation).

Imaging

- If the diagnosis is equivocal after history-taking, physical examination, and handheld Doppler evaluation, ultrasound is the first-line study to confirm the diagnosis. Color Doppler shows a poorly defined hypervascular lesion with fast-flow and shunting. A parenchymal mass is not present.

- Tortuous feeding arteries are visualized, with dilated draining veins and significant flow.
- Arteriovenous malformation can be differentiated from hemangioma because hemangioma has parenchymal tissue.
- MRI is usually obtained to confirm the diagnosis, determine the extent of the lesion, and plan treatment.
- Images are obtained with contrast and fat suppression. Arteriovenous malformations exhibit dilated feeding arteries/draining veins, enhancement, and flow-voids. Unlike hemangioma, arteriovenous malformation does not have a parenchymal mass. MR angiography shows feeding arterial vessels and early enhancement of draining veins (Fig. 12-4).

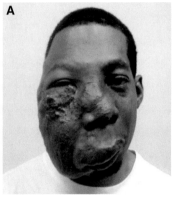
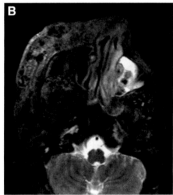
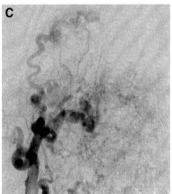

Fig. 12-4 **A,** This 28-year-old man has a diffuse stage III lesion involving the right side of the face causing ulceration, pain, and bleeding. **B,** Axial MRI shows diffuse signal abnormality, with flow-voids and overgrowth of the right side of his face. **C,** Angiogram shows a large nidus with early filling of draining veins because of shunting.

- An angiogram is obtained if the diagnosis remains unclear after ultrasound and MRI, or if embolization is planned. Angiography shows the flow dynamics of the lesion and identifies the tortuous or dilated arteries, the enlarged draining veins, and the nidus. The nidus contains tortuous small vessels with ill-defined vascular spaces.
- CT may be indicated if an arteriovenous malformation involves bone.

Histopathology

- Histopathologic diagnosis of arteriovenous malformation is rarely necessary. A biopsy is indicated only if imaging is equivocal or if a malignancy is suspected.
- Biopsy of an arteriovenous malformation may be complicated by bleeding and growth of the lesion.
- Large, tortuous arteries with thin- and thick-walled veins are present. Arteries may have disrupted internal elastic lamina (demonstrated by Verhoeff-van Gieson staining). Veins have thickened muscular walls that become fibrotic, causing a thin, inelastic structure. Intimal and adventitial fibrosis occurs. Areas may have a small vessel component which contains proliferating endothelial cells and pericytes.
- *PTEN*-AVA shows features typical of an arteriovenous malformation (tortuous vessels with arterialized veins). In addition, *PTEN*-AVA has significant fibromyxoid areas, adipose tissue, and lymphoid clusters. Arteries have transmural muscular hyperplasia and small lumens. Very thin−walled veins can appear similar to pulmonary alveoli.

MANAGEMENT

Nonoperative Treatment

- Hydrated petroleum should be placed over superficial arteriovenous malformations to prevent desiccation, incidental trauma to the skin, and subsequent ulceration.
- Compression garments for extremity lesions may reduce pain and swelling.
- Bleeding is controlled by compression and further intervention is rarely necessary.
- Because estrogen is proangiogenic and theoretically may stimulate arteriovenous malformation progression, estrogen-containing contraceptives should be avoided.
- Although pregnancy has been thought to increase the risk of arteriovenous malformation expansion, pregnant women with stage I lesions do not have an increased rate of progression compared with women who are not pregnant. However, pregnancy in women with a stage II through IV arteriovenous malformation has not been studied, and thus women with advanced lesions should be cautioned that pregnancy may exacerbate the malformation.
- Drugs for arteriovenous malformation currently do not exist; however, oral thalidomide might reduce symptoms and vascularity in patients with stage III and IV arteriovenous malformations.

Timing of Intervention

- Arteriovenous malformation is not a malignancy and intervention is not mandatory.
- Management is focused on alleviating symptoms (such as bleeding, pain, ulceration), preserving vital functions (such as vision, mastication), and improving a deformity.
- Treatment options include embolization, sclerotherapy, and/or resection.

- 75% of patients require intervention in childhood or adolescence. The remaining individuals do not need treatment until adulthood.
- The goal of management usually is to control the arteriovenous malformation. Because the lesion is often diffuse and involves multiple tissue planes, cure is rare.
- An asymptomatic arteriovenous malformation should be observed unless it can be removed for possible cure with minimal morbidity. Embolization or incomplete excision of an asymptomatic lesion may stimulate it to enlarge and become problematic.
- Intervention is determined by the size and location of the arteriovenous malformation, age of the patient, and Schobinger stage.
- Although resection of an asymptomatic stage I arteriovenous malformation offers the best chance for long-term control or cure, intervention must be individualized based on the degree of deformity that would be caused by excision and reconstruction. For example, a stage I arteriovenous malformation in a location that is not anatomically important, such as the trunk, may be easily resected before it progresses to a higher stage, when excision would be more difficult and the likelihood of recurrence greater.
- In contrast, a large, asymptomatic arteriovenous malformation on the face is best observed, especially in a young child not psychologically prepared for a major procedure. Resection and reconstruction may result in a more noticeable deformity or functional problem than the malformation.
- Although the recurrence rate is lower when a stage I arteriovenous malformation is resected, it is still high, and thus even after major resection and reconstruction the malformation may recur.
- Some children (17.4%) do not experience significant morbidity from their arteriovenous malformation until they are adults.
- Intervention for a stage II arteriovenous malformation is similar to that for a stage I lesion, although the threshold for treatment is lower if an enlarging lesion is causing a worsening deformity or if functional problems are expected.
- Stage III and IV arteriovenous malformations require intervention to control pain, bleeding, ulceration, or heart failure.

Embolization

- Embolization is the delivery of a substance through an arterial catheter to occlude blood flow and/or fill a vascular space. Success requires that the embolic agent reach the nidus of the arteriovenous malformation at the point of initial venous drainage.
- In addition to the replacement of arterialized blood with an inert embolic substance, ischemia and scarring further reduce arteriovenous shunting, shrink the lesion, and improve symptoms.
- Embolization is not curative, and most arteriovenous malformations will reexpand after treatment. Even if significant volume reduction does not occur, symptoms are improved. Indications for embolization include preoperative intervention to reduce blood loss during resection (Fig. 12-5) or definitive treatment to alleviate symptoms for lesions not amenable to resection.

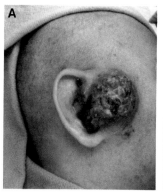
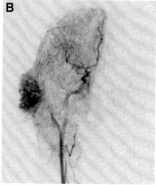
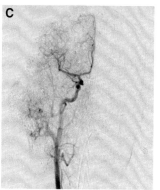

Fig. 12-5   Embolization of arteriovenous malformation. **A,** A 15-year-old boy with a stage III AVM causing ulceration, bleeding, and pain. **B,** An angiogram illustrates a nidus, arteriovenous shunting, and early filling of draining veins. **C,** After preoperative embolization, angiography shows nonopacification of the nidus and reduced shunting.

- Proximal arterial embolization is contraindicated because recanalization occurs and the lesion becomes inaccessible for future embolization.
- Embolization typically is performed under general anesthesia and multiple treatments every 6 weeks are usually required.
- Because the arteriovenous malformation is not removed, almost all lesions eventually will reexpand after treatment. Multiple embolizations do not lower the rate of recurrence, although newer embolic agents (such as Onyx) may offer more lasting results.
- A stage I arteriovenous malformation has a lower recurrence rate than higher-staged lesions. Most recurrences occur within the first year after embolization, and 98% reexpand within 5 years (although newer embolic agents may be more efficacious).
- Patients who have not exhibited enlargement 5 years after embolization are more likely to have long-term control.
- Despite the high risk of reexpansion, embolization can effectively palliate an arteriovenous malformation by alleviating pain and bleeding.
- Embolization is typically performed before a planned resection to reduce blood loss during the extirpation.
- Substances used for embolization may be liquid (N-butyl cyanoacrylate, Onyx, or ethanol) or solid (polyvinyl alcohol particles or coils).
- The choice of embolic agent depends on whether embolization is being used as primary treatment or as a preoperative adjunct to excision. For preoperative embolization, temporary occlusive substances (Gelfoam powder, polyvinyl alcohol particles, embospheres) are used.
- Delivery of polyvinyl alcohol particles and embospheres with different particle sizes allows the initial occlusion of small, distal vessels followed by blockage of more proximal branches with larger emboli.
- Permanent liquid agents capable of permeating the nidus (ethanol, N-butyl cyanoacrylate, Onyx) are more often used when embolization is the primary treatment.

- We prefer Onyx for both primary treatment and preoperative embolization. Onyx is an ethylene-vinyl alcohol copolymer that precipitates on the surface after contacting blood. A liquid core is maintained that allows the injection of multiple nidal areas. Onyx allows more aggressive embolization than other liquid agents.
- The most frequent complication of embolization is ulceration, which is more common for superficial lesions. Wounds are allowed to heal secondarily.
- Distal migration of embolic material can cause ischemic injury to uninvolved tissues. Unlike sclerotherapy for slow-flow vascular malformations, posttreatment edema after embolization of an arteriovenous malformation is less severe (unless ethanol is used as the embolic agent).
- Most patients are observed overnight in the hospital. Posttreatment swelling may necessitate close monitoring if an airway or orbital arteriovenous malformation is treated.
- Deep extremity lesions are at risk for compartment syndrome.
- Patients and families are counseled that an arteriovenous malformation is likely to reexpand after treatment, and thus additional embolizations may be required in the future.

Sclerotherapy

- Sclerotherapy is the transcutaneous injection of a substance into the malformation, which causes endothelial destruction and thrombosis. Fibrosis of the vascular space decreases the size of the lesion and improves symptoms.
- Indications for sclerotherapy include a well-localized arteriovenous malformation, occlusion of veins draining the arteriovenous malformation, and an arteriovenous malformation that cannot be accessed transarterially, usually because previous embolization has occluded the feeding arteries.
- Our preferred sclerosants are sodium tetradecyl sulfate (STS) and ethanol. Although ethanol is more effective than sodium tetradecyl sulfate, it has a higher complication rate.

- Because ethanol can cause nerve damage, it should be used cautiously in proximity to important structures, such as the facial nerve. The dose should not exceed 1 ml/kg (maximum 60 ml).
- Sclerotherapy of an arteriovenous malformation presents a higher risk than treatment of a slow-flow lesion, because the sclerosant is more likely to escape into the systemic circulation.

Operative Treatment

- Resection of an arteriovenous malformation has a lower recurrence rate than embolization. Indications include a well-localized lesion, correction of a focal deformity (such as bleeding or ulcerated areas, labial hypertrophy), or a symptomatic arteriovenous malformation that has failed embolization (Fig. 12-6).
- Extirpation and reconstruction of a large, diffuse arteriovenous malformation should be exercised with caution because cure is rare and the recurrence rate is high, the resulting deformity is often worse than the appearance of the malformation, and resection is associated with significant blood loss, iatrogenic injury, and morbidity.
- When excision is planned, preoperative embolization will facilitate the procedure by minimizing blood loss. Excision should be carried out 24 to 72 hours after embolization, before recanalization and neovascularization restores blood flow to the lesion, especially if temporary agents are used. If Onyx is the embolic material, resection can be performed up to 14 days after the embolization.
- To reduce blood loss, an epinephrine-containing local anesthetic is infused throughout the operative field and a tourniquet is used when removing an extremity lesion.
- Small, well-localized arteriovenous malformations or those that cannot be accessed for embolization may be resected without preoperative embolization.
- Proximal feeding vessels to the arteriovenous malformation should never be ligated because collateralization will stimulate enlargement, and access for future embolization will no longer be possible.

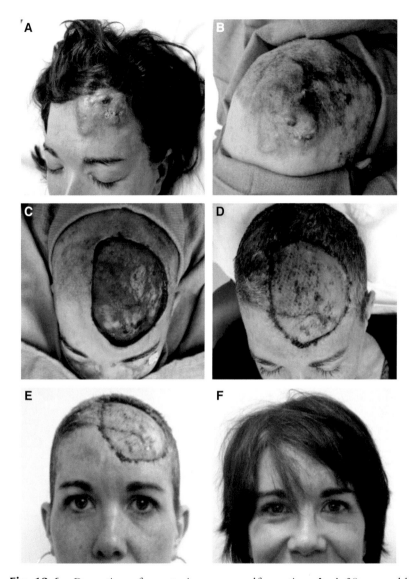

Fig. 12-6 Resection of an arteriovenous malformation. **A,** A 39-year-old woman with an ulcerated, bleeding, painful stage III AVM of the forehead and scalp. **B,** Intraoperative view after preoperative embolization. **C,** Soft tissue defect after resection. **D** and **E,** The wound was closed using a split-thickness skin graft. **F,** Nine months postoperatively, the graft is concealed by hair.

- Surgical margins are best determined clinically by assessing the amount of bleeding from the wound edges. Frozen section analysis of margins is not reliable.
- Most defects can be reconstructed by advancing local skin flaps.
- Skin grafting ulcerated areas has a high failure rate because the underlying tissue is ischemic. Excision with regional flap transfer may be required.
- Free-flap reconstruction permits wide resection and primary closure of complicated defects. Although it has been proposed that free tissue transfer may minimize recurrence by reducing hypoxia, free-tissue transfer does not improve long–term arteriovenous malformation control.
- Despite subtotal and presumed complete extirpation, most arteriovenous malformations treated by resection recur. Serial excisions do not reduce the recurrence rate.
- Most recurrences occur within the first year after resection, and 86% reexpand within 5 years. Patients who have not exhibited recurrence 5 years after excision are likely to achieve long-term control, although 5% of lesions will reexpand more than 10 years later.
- Patients and families are counseled that the arteriovenous malformation is likely to recur after resection, and thus intervention may be required in the future.

Selected References

Alomari AI, Chaudry G, Rodesch G, Burrows PE, Mulliken JB, Smith ER, Fishman SJ, Orbach DB. Complex spinal-paraspinal fast-flow lesions in CLOVES syndrome: analysis of clinical and imaging findings in 6 patients. AJNR Am J Neuroradiol 32:1812-1817, 2011.

Arnold R, Chaudry G. Diagnostic imaging of vascular anomalies. Clin Plast Surg 38:21-29, 2011.

Eerola I, Boon LM, Mulliken JB, Burrows PE, Dompmartin A, Watanabe S, Vanwijck R, Vikkula M. Capillary malformation-arteriovenous malformation: a new clinical and genetic disorder caused by RASA1 mutations. Am J Hum Genet 73:1240-1249, 2003.

Greene AK, Orbach DB. Management of arteriovenous malformations. Clin Plast Surg 38:95-106, 2011.

Gupta A, Kozakewich H. Histopathology of vascular anomalies. Clin Plast Surg 38:31-44, 2011.

Liu AS, Mulliken JB, Zurakowski D, Fishman SJ, Greene AK. Extracranial arteriovenous malformations: natural progression and recurrence after treatment. Plast Reconstr Surg 125:1185-1194, 2011.

McDonald J, Bayrak-Toydemir P, Ryeritz RE. Hereditary hemorrhagic telangiectasia: an overview of diagnosis, management, and pathogenesis. Genet Med 13:607-616, 2011.

Mulliken JB, Fishman SJ, Burrows PE. Vascular anomalies. Curr Prob Surg 37:517-584, 2000.

Revencu N, Boon LM, Mulliken JB, Enjolras O, Cordisco MR, Burrows PE, Clapuyt P, Hammer F, Dubois J, Baselga E, Brancati F, Carder R, Quintal JM, Dallapiccola B, Fischer G, Frieden IJ, Garzon M, Harper J, Johnson-Patel J, Labrèze C, Martorell L, Paltiel HJ, Pohl A, Prendiville J, Quere I, Siegel DH, Valente EM, Van Hagen A, Van Hest L, Vaux KK, Vicente A, Weibel L, Chitayat D, Vikkula M. Parkes Weber syndrome, vein of Galen aneurysmal malformation, and other fast-flow vascular anomalies are caused by RASA1 mutations. Hum Mutat 29:959-965, 2008.

Schmidt D, Pache M, Schumacher M. The congenital unilateral retino-cephalic vascular malformation syndrome (Bonnet-Dechaume-Blanc syndrome or Wyburn-Mason syndrome): review of the literature. Surv Ophthalmol 53:227-249, 2008.

Tan WH, Baris HN, Burrows PE, Robson CD, Alomari AI, Mulliken JB, Fishman SJ, Irons MB. The spectrum of vascular anomalies in patients with PTEN mutations: implications for diagnosis and management. J Med Genet 44:594-602, 2007.

Thiex R, Mulliken JB, Revencu N, Boon LM, Burrows PE, Cordisco M, Dwight Y, Smith ER, Vikkula M, Orbach DB. A novel association between RASA1 mutations and spinal arteriovenous anomalies. AJNR Am J Neuroradiol 31:775-779, 2010.

Thiex R, Wu I, Mulliken JB, Greene AK, Rahbar R, Orbach D. Safety and efficacy of onyx embolization for extracranial head and neck and vascular anomalies. AJNR Am J Neuroradiol 32:1082-1086, 2011.

Wu IC, Orbach DB. Neurointerventional management of high-flow vascular malformations of the head and neck. Neuroimag Clin N Am 19:219-240, 2009.

CHAPTER 13

Vascular Malformation Overgrowth Syndromes

TUMORS	MALFORMATIONS		
	Slow-Flow	**Fast-Flow**	**Overgrowth Syndromes**
Infantile Hemangioma	*Capillary Malformation*	*Arteriovenous Malformation*	CLOVES Klippel-Trenaunay Maffucci Parkes Weber Proteus Sturge-Weber
Congenital Hemangioma	*Lymphatic Malformation*		
Kaposiform Hemangioendothelioma	*Venous Malformation*		
Pyogenic Granuloma			
Rare Vascular Tumors			

CLOVES SYNDROME

CLINICAL FEATURES

- CLOVES is an acronym for *c*ongenital *l*ipomatosis, *o*vergrowth, *v*ascular malformations, *e*pidermal nevi, and *s*coliosis/*s*keletal/ *s*pinal anomalies (Fig. 13-1).
- The condition is nonfamilial and is caused by a somatic mosaic activating mutation in *PIK3CA*.
- Males and females are affected equally.
- Many of these patients previously were thought to have Proteus syndrome. Two major features distinguish CLOVES syndrome from Proteus syndrome:
  - Patients with CLOVES syndrome do not have cerebriform connective tissue nevi involving the hands or feet.
  - Proteus syndrome is significantly progressive.
- All patients with CLOVES syndrome have a truncal lipomatous mass (usually over the posterolateral back or flank), a slow-flow vascular malformation (typically a capillary malformation overlying the lipomatous mass), and hand or foot anomalies (increased width, macrodactyly, first web space "sandal gap").
- Common features include paraspinal fast-flow malformations, linear epidermal nevi, and hemihypertrophy. Less frequent associated conditions include neurologic anomalies, such as neural tube defect or tethered cord, and renal agenesis or hypoplasia.
- The lipomatous masses typically cause pain and can infiltrate adjacent areas, such as the retroperitoneum, mediastinum, paraspinal muscles, and epidural space.

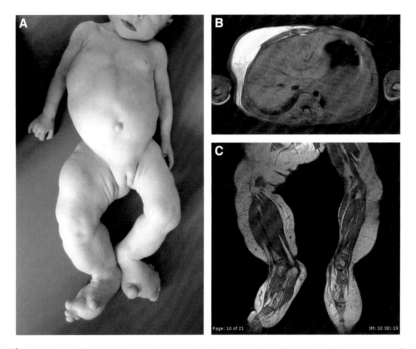

Fig. 13-1   CLOVES syndrome. **A,** A 6-month-old girl with overgrowth of the lower extremities, foot anomalies, and lipomatous masses of the trunk. **B,** An axial T1 MR image shows an anterior truncal lipomatous mass. **C,** A coronal T1 MR sequence shows adipose overgrowth of the lower extremities.

- Vascular malformations consist of:
  - Capillary malformations usually involving the skin above the lipomatous mass
  - Lymphatic malformations within the truncal lipomatous masses (83%)
  - Arteriovenous malformations within or around lipomatous masses in the paraspinal area (28%)
  - Venous malformations (phlebectasia) involving the truncal lesions (16%)
- Central and thoracic phlebectasia can cause perioperative pulmonary embolism and thus thromboembolism prophylaxis should be employed before a surgical intervention.
- Musculoskeletal anomalies include:
  - Wide triangular feet, large hands, macrodactyly (usually the middle toe or finger)
  - A widened sandal gap (typically the first web space of the foot)
  - Scoliosis
- The truncal masses are predominantly lipomatous tissue that may contain a lymphatic component.

DIAGNOSIS

Imaging

- MRI is obtained to determine whether the spinal cord is threatened by a lipomatous lesion or arteriovenous malformation. MRI also delineates whether thoracic phlebectasia is present that may predispose the patient to a thromboembolic event.
- Affected children are at risk for developing Wilms tumor; therefore they require renal ultrasound examination every 3 months until they reach 8 years of age.

Histopathology

- Histopathology is nonspecific for CLOVES syndrome; the diagnosis is made by physical examination.
- Biopsy is indicated if a malignancy is suspected, such as Wilms tumor.

MANAGEMENT

- Resection of a subcutaneous lipomatous mass is indicated only to alleviate pain or improve a deformity. The recurrence rate is very high and almost all patients have some regrowth of the lesion.
- Paraspinal arteriovenous malformations may require embolization or resection to prevent spinal cord ischemia. Lipomatous lesions involving the spinal cord may necessitate resection.
- Lymphatic and venous malformations may benefit from sclerotherapy, and capillary malformations can be improved with pulsed-dye laser.
- An orthopedic consultation is obtained to determine whether a leg-length discrepancy is present. Patients may require amputations or soft tissue debulking to facilitate ambulation.
- Hand surgery consultation is obtained if significant musculoskeletal hand anomalies might be improved with operative intervention.

KLIPPEL-TRENAUNAY SYNDROME

CLINICAL FEATURES

• Klippel-Trenaunay syndrome (KTS) is a capillary-lymphatic-venous malformation (CLVM) of an extremity causing soft tissue and/or skeletal overgrowth (Fig. 13-2).

• There is tremendous phenotypic variability, from a slightly enlarged extremity with a capillary stain to a massively overgrown limb with malformed digits. In 10% of patients the involved extremity is hypoplastic.

• The condition almost always affects the lower limb (95%); upper extremity involvement is rare (5%).

• The contralateral foot or hand may be enlarged and will exhibit macrodactyly.

• The capillary malformation is typically distributed over the lateral side of the extremity, buttock, or thorax. It is macular in a neonate, and over time lymphatic vesicles can develop in the stain.

• Pelvic involvement is common with lower extremity disease and can cause hematuria, bladder outlet obstruction, cystitis, and hematochezia.

• Upper extremity or truncal disease can affect the posterior mediastinum and retropleural space.

• The venous component of Klippel-Trenaunay syndrome manifests as phlebectasia and abnormal drainage of the affected area.

• A large embryonic vein in the subcutaneous tissue (the marginal vein of Servelle) is isolated in the lateral calf or thigh and communicates with the deep venous system. Complications include thrombophlebitis (20% to 45%) and pulmonary embolism (4% to 24%).

• The lymphatic abnormalities are usually macrocystic in the pelvis/thigh and microcystic in the abdominal wall, buttock, and distal limb.

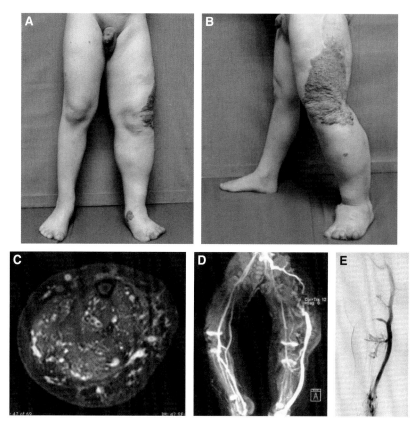

Fig. 13-2   Klippel-Trenaunay syndrome. **A** and **B,** A 6-year-old boy with a capillary-venous-lymphatic malformation of the left lower extremity causing overgrowth. **C,** An axial MR image shows a diffuse vascular malformation involving tissues above and below the muscle fascia. **D,** A coronal MR venogram reveals a lateral embryonic vein. **E,** Venography delineates the anatomy of the marginal vein of Servelle.

DIAGNOSIS

Imaging

- An MRI is obtained to confirm the diagnosis, determine the extent of disease, and plan treatment.
- The MRI shows soft tissue and often bony overgrowth. Lymphatic and venous malformations are noted. Venous components typically enhance with contrast and involve muscle. Lymphatic anomalies are usually infiltrative and do not enhance significantly. An important feature of Klippel-Trenaunay syndrome is that the tissues above and below the muscle fascia are affected by the malformation. In contrast, other causes of extremity overgrowth only involve the area above the muscle fascia (for example, lymphedema, capillary malformation, and lipedema).
- The embryonic marginal vein of Servelle is pathognomonic for Klippel-Trenaunay syndrome. It is a dilated vein that travels in the subcutis along the lateral calf and thigh.
- Treatment may be based on the MRI results, depending on the relative contributions of the venous or lymphatic anomalies.

Histopathology

- Histopathology is not specific for Klippel-Trenaunay syndrome; thus biopsy is not indicated for diagnosis.
- Histopathologic examination shows capillary, venous, and/or lymphatic malformation, depending on the area of the limb where the tissue was resected.

MANAGEMENT

- Orthopedic consultation is necessary to monitor for a leg-length discrepancy and to determine whether selective amputations are needed to facilitate footwear and ambulation. By 2 years of age, surveillance of leg-length by plain radiography is indicated. If the discrepancy is more than 1.5 cm, a shoe-lift for the shorter limb can prevent limping and scoliosis. Epiphysiodesis of the distal femoral growth plate is typically done at about 11 years of age. Enlargement of the foot may require a ray, midfoot, or Syme amputation to allow the use of footwear.
- Unlike some other overgrowth conditions, such as isolated hemihypertrophy or CLOVES syndrome, patients with Klippel-Trenaunay syndrome are not at increased risk for the development of Wilms tumor, and screening is unnecessary.
- Venous anomalies are managed with compression garments for insufficiency and aspirin to minimize phlebothrombosis. Symptomatic varicose veins may be removed or sclerosed. Because embryonal veins can connect to the deep venous system causing thromboembolism, they are removed in early childhood with sclerotherapy or endovascular laser. Venous insufficiency of the extremity does not occur following removal of the large superficial embryonal vein, because a functioning deep venous system is present. The deep system is often difficult to visualize on imaging because of predominant flow in the superficial veins. After removal of the lateral embryonal vein of Servelle, the deep venous system dilates and is more easily seen radiographically.
- Lymphatic anomalies are treated by sclerotherapy if they are macrocystic. Bleeding and/or oozing cutaneous microcystic vesicles are managed by sclerotherapy, carbon dioxide laser, or resection (large areas may require excision and skin grafting).
- Circumferential overgrowth can be improved with staged skin and subcutaneous resection. Venous insufficiency does not occur after excision, because a deep venous system is present.

MAFFUCCI SYNDROME

CLINICAL FEATURES

- Maffucci syndrome is a nonhereditary disorder characterized by multiple enchondromas (benign tumor of chondrocytes) and soft tissue vascular lesions (Fig. 13-3).
- The disease affects all races and does not have a sex predominance. Patients have normal intelligence.
- Maffucci syndrome is one of seven enchondromatosis syndromes (subtype 2), and is similar to Ollier disease (subtype 1), except that it also has soft tissue vascular anomalies.
- The condition is caused by a somatic mosaic mutation in isocitrate dehydrogenase (IDH); 77% of patients have a lesion with a mutation in either *IDH1* (98%) or *IDH2* (2%).
- The average age at presentation is 4 years; 27% of patients are diagnosed at birth, and 78% present before puberty.
- The soft tissue vascular anomaly is called a *spindle cell hemangioma,* but this lesion is probably a reactive process in an underlying venous malformation. Clinically, the vascular anomaly is most consistent with a venous malformation because it is blue, can be emptied with pressure or elevation, and contains phleboliths.
- The spindle cell hemangioma or venous malformation can affect the hand (57%), foot (41%), arm (39%), leg (38%), trunk (29%), and head or neck (25%). It has also been reported in the viscera and mucous membranes.
- The vascular lesions can cause overgrowth of the affected area, pain from phlebothrombosis, and limitation of function, especially if the hand is involved.
- Enchondromas most commonly involve the hands (89%), followed by the tibia/fibula (52%), foot (36%), femur (36%), humerus (34%), radius/ulna (29%), ribs (27%), pelvis (25%), scapula (20%), and head (18%).
- The enchondromas are within bone (endosteal) and can cause progressive skeletal deformity, such as bowing, shortening of ex-

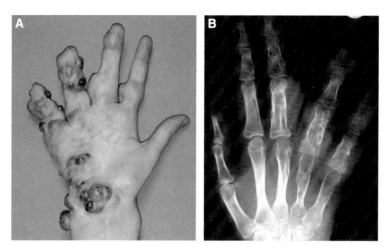

Fig. 13-3   Maffucci syndrome. **A,** A 16-year-old girl with multiple vascular lesions (spindle cell hemangiomas/venous malformations) involving the right hand. **B,** Plain radiography shows multiple enchondromas of the hand.

tremities, leg-length discrepancy, and scoliosis. Pathologic fractures affect 26% of patients.
- The risk of chondrosarcoma forming in an underlying enchondroma is 15% to 30%. The average age is 40 years (range 13 to 69 years). Most chondrosarcomas are grade 1 (58%), 36% are grade 2, and 6% are grade 3.
- Enchondromas involving the small bones of the hands or feet have a 14% risk of malignant transformation. Lesions affecting the long bones of the extremities or axial skeleton have a greater chance of progression to chondrosarcoma (44% to 50%). Patients with enchondromas of the pelvis have a 3.8 times higher risk of developing chondrosarcoma in any area.
- In addition to chondrosarcoma, patients with Maffucci syndrome are at risk for developing additional tumors, most commonly brain, hepatic, pancreatic, and ovarian, or acute myeloid leukemia. Sarcomas have been documented to arise from the soft tissue vascular lesions.

- The disease can be fatal because of pulmonary metastasis from a chondrosarcoma, although the most common cause of death is a noncartilaginous tumor (for example, brain, liver, pancreas, ovary, angiosarcoma).

DIAGNOSIS

Imaging

- All patients with suspected Maffucci syndrome undergo conventional radiography to confirm the disease tumor (if enchondromas are present) and rule out a bony malignancy.
- On plain radiography, enchondromas are intramedullary (central). They appear as radiolucent lesions with osseous expansile remodeling and cortical thinning. Enchondromas do not cause cortical destruction or soft tissue extension. Soft tissue phleboliths in the vascular lesions often are present.
- For patients with suspected Maffucci syndrome, conventional radiographs are taken to define the baseline appearance of all enchondromas. Screening radiographs are subsequently obtained to assess for malignant changes, such as new or progressive cortical destruction or soft tissue extension. The onset of pain, swelling, or neurologic findings also mandates imaging.
- If possible malignant transformation of an enchondroma is noted on plain radiography, an MRI of the area is obtained.
- Patients with head or abdominal complaints undergo CT or MRI to rule out a possible malignancy of the brain or viscera.

Histopathology

- Histopathology is nondiagnostic for Maffucci syndrome. Patients are identified by physical examination findings of soft tissue vascular lesions and radiographic evidence of multiple enchondromas.
- A biopsy is indicated if malignant transformation of an enchondroma is suspected clinically and supported by imaging.

- Enchondromas appear as lobules of hyaline and myxoid chondroid matrix, with enchondral ossification of the matrix. Cytonuclear atypia and mitotic figures are not present.
- The soft tissue vascular anomaly associated with Maffucci syndrome is called a *spindle cell hemangioma*. This lesion is likely a reactive response inside a venous malformation and is considered a malformation rather than a tumor. Lesions consist of thin-walled venous spaces, spindled fibroblasts, and cellular areas with collapsed vessels. Phleboliths are present. The endothelium can appear epithelioid and have cytoplasmic vacuolization. Atypia and mitosis are not present.

MANAGEMENT

- Orthopedic intervention is based on symptoms, such as limited function, pain, scoliosis, or leg-length discrepancy.
- Problematic enchondromas are treated by curettage or excision and bone grafting.
- Chondrosarcomas are managed based on grade. Low-grade tumors can be treated by resection or curettage with or without adjuvant therapy, including phenol, ethanol, or cryosurgery. Higher-grade lesions are managed by resection or amputation. Chemotherapy and radiotherapy are not effective.
- Soft tissue spindle cell hemangioma or venous malformation can be treated with sclerotherapy and/or resection if symptoms are present, such as pain or inhibited function.
- A recent report showed a reduction in the size of soft tissue vascular lesions and improved symptoms in a patient with Maffucci syndrome treated with sirolimus.

PARKES WEBER SYNDROME

CLINICAL FEATURES

- Parkes Weber syndrome (PWS) consists of a diffuse arteriovenous malformation of an extremity causing soft tissue and/or bony overgrowth. A capillary malformation involves the skin of the affected limb. The condition most commonly involves one lower extremity (Fig. 13-4).
- The malformation is evident at birth. The limb exhibits symmetrical enlargement, and the cutaneous stain is warmer than a typical capillary malformation.

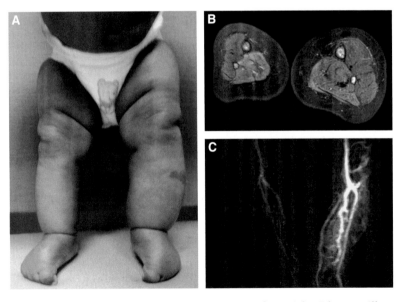

Fig. 13-4   Parkes Weber syndrome. **A,** An infant girl with a capillary-arteriovenous malformation of the left lower extremity causing limb overgrowth. **B,** An axial T2 MR image shows enlargement of all structures of the leg, including the muscle compartment. **C,** An MR angiogram illustrates enlarged arterial inflow to the extremity.

- Parkes Weber syndrome can be sporadic or familial as a result of a mutation in *RASA1* (capillary malformation–arteriovenous malformation).
- Parkes Weber syndrome caused by a *RASA1* mutation can affect an upper limb (in a third of affected individuals) or a lower extremity (in two thirds). The overlying capillary malformation is heterogenous—single, multiple, localized, or diffuse.
- *RASA1* mutations have not been found in patients with Parkes Weber syndrome who do not have multifocal capillary malformations.
- The diagnosis is confirmed by the detection of a bruit or thrill. Handheld Doppler examination reveals that fast-flow is present.
- Patients have subcutaneous and intramuscular microshunting and can develop symptomatic congestive heart failure (6%).

DIAGNOSIS

Imaging

- An MRI is obtained to confirm the diagnosis and determine the extent of the malformation. All components of the extremity are typically overgrown—subcutis, muscle, and bone. Diffuse microfistulas are seen as flow-voids. The enlarged limb muscles and bones show abnormal signal and enhancement.
- MR angiography and venography exhibit dilated, tortuous arteries and draining veins.
- Ultrasound shows fast-flow and shunting.
- Angiography demonstrates discrete arteriovenous shunts.

Histopathology

- Histopathology is not specific for Parkes Weber syndrome; the diagnosis is made by history, physical examination, and imaging.
- Histopathology shows arteriovenous or capillary malformation, depending on the area of the limb from which the tissue was harvested.

MANAGEMENT

- Most children are observed until symptoms necessitate intervention.
- In rare instances, an infant presents with high-output congestive heart failure caused by shunting through arteriovenous fistulas. Embolization to reduce shunting is performed with permanent occlusive agents. Repeated embolizations are often necessary.
- Children are monitored annually by an orthopedic surgeon for axial overgrowth. By 2 years of age, radiologic surveillance of leg length by plain radiography is indicated. If the discrepancy is more than 1.5 cm, a shoe-lift for the shorter limb can prevent limping and scoliosis. Epiphysiodesis of the distal femoral growth plate is typically performed around 11 years of age.
- Embolization may be useful for pain or cutaneous ischemic changes. Occasionally, amputation is necessary.
- Patients with Parkes Weber syndrome should be followed by a cardiologist to monitor for signs of congestive heart failure.
- Patients should be tested for the presence of a *RASA1* mutation (especially if the child has multifocal capillary malformations or a family history of capillary malformations/arteriovenous malformations). If a *RASA1* mutation is present, an MRI is obtained to rule out brain and/or spinal arteriovenous malformations. The patient and family are also counseled about the autosomal dominant transmission of the mutation.

PROTEUS SYNDROME

CLINICAL FEATURES

- Proteus syndrome is a sporadic overgrowth disorder caused by a somatic mosaic activating mutation in *AKT1* (Fig. 13-5).
- Approximately 100 cases have been documented, and males are more commonly affected (2:1).

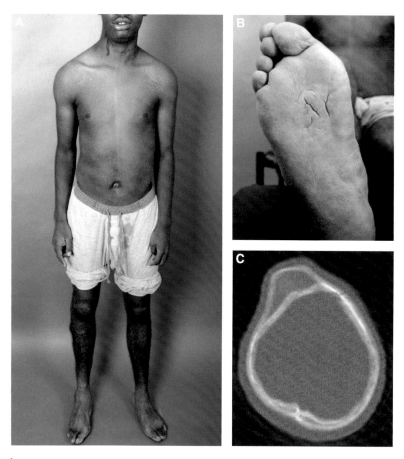

Fig. 13-5   Proteus syndrome. **A,** An 18-year-old boy with progressive skeletal overgrowth of the right lower extremity requiring epiphysiodesis; adipose overgrowth of the trunk; venous malformations of the right lower limb; scoliosis; epidermal nevi of the face and neck; anomalous optic nerves; and developmental delay. **B,** Cerebriform nevus of the plantar foot. **C,** Hyperostosis of the cranium.

- The major features of Proteus syndrome are:
  - Progressive, asymmetrical, disproportionate overgrowth of body parts (typically skeletal/limbs)
  - Cerebriform connective tissue nevi (the palmar aspect of the hands, the plantar surface of the feet, the chest)
  - Epidermal nevi (50%)
  - Vascular malformations (capillary, venous, lymphatic)
  - Adipose overgrowth
  - Cerebral anomalies (40%) (developmental delay, seizures, malformations)
  - Ophthalmologic findings (40%) (strabismus, epibulbar cysts, epibulbar dermoids)
  - Cystic lung disease (9%)
  - Renal/urologic anomalies (9%)
  - Bone disorders (skull hyperostoses, megaspondylodysplasia)
- The significant progression of the disease and the cerebriform connective tissue nevus are pathognomonic for the syndrome.
- A facial phenotype is common: dolichocephaly, a long face, down-slanting palpebral fissures or ptosis, a low nasal bridge, wide or anteverted nares, an open mouth at rest.
- Patients have a 20% mortality rate from venous thrombosis/pulmonary embolism, cystic lung disease, and neoplasms.
- Individuals are at high risk for deep venous thrombosis because of vascular malformations, immobility, and surgical procedures.
- The most common tumors associated with Proteus syndrome are ovarian cystadenoma, meningioma, testicular tumor, and parotid adenoma.
- The primary differential diagnosis is CLOVES syndrome. Patients with Proteus syndrome (unlike CLOVES syndrome) have (1) significantly progressive overgrowth and (2) cerebriform connective tissue nevus (usually hands and feet). The two syndromes can now be differentiated genetically because they are caused by different somatic mutations (Proteus = *AKT1;* CLOVES = *PIK3CA*).

DIAGNOSIS

Imaging

- A CT and/or an MRI is obtained to evaluate for pulmonary cystic lesions, intraabdominal lipomas, and central nervous system anomalies.
- Skeletal radiographs are used to rule out megaspondylodysplasia or vertebral body asymmetry.

Histopathology

- Histopathology is nonspecific for Proteus syndrome; the diagnosis is made by history and clinical examination.
- A biopsy is indicated if a malignancy is suspected.

MANAGEMENT

- Neurology, ophthalmology, and pulmonology consultations are obtained.
- Patients usually require orthopedic intervention for skeletal morbidity (for example, epiphysiodesis, joint replacement, and spinal fusion).
- Problematic venous and lymphatic malformations are treated by sclerotherapy and/or resection.
- Antithrombotic prophylaxis is administered if an operative procedure is planned.

STURGE-WEBER SYNDROME

CLINICAL FEATURES

- Sturge–Weber syndrome (SWS) is a sporadic neurocutaneous disorder that affects 1/50,000 newborns.
- The syndrome is defined by a capillary malformation in the V_1 trigeminal nerve distribution (forehead/eyelid) with either ocular abnormalities (glaucoma, choroidal vascular anomalies) and/or a leptomeningeal vascular malformation (Fig. 13-6).
- The capillary malformation can be in the ophthalmic (V_1), extend into the maxillary (V_2), or involve all three trigeminal dermatomes. Patients with maxillary or mandibular involvement alone are at low risk for Sturge–Weber syndrome.
- Patients also commonly have soft tissue and/or bony overgrowth (60% to 83%); the frequency is similar to the risk for glaucoma (65% to 77%) and for neurologic problems (87% to 93%).
- The leptomeningeal anomalies may be capillary, venous, or arteriovenous malformations. Small foci can be silent, but extensive pial vascular lesions may cause refractory seizures, contralateral hemiplegia, and/or delayed motor and cognitive development. Patients with bilateral facial capillary malformations have a higher risk of brain anomalies.
- The anomalous choroidal vascularity can cause retinal detachment, glaucoma, and blindness.
- In addition to the facial capillary malformation, patients often have generalized extracraniofacial capillary malformations (29%). When a diffuse extremity stain is present, patients with Sturge–Weber syndrome have been erroneously labeled as having Klippel–Weber–Trenaunay syndrome, Klippel–Trenaunay syndrome, or Parkes Weber syndrome. In contrast to Klippel–Trenaunay or Parkes Weber syndromes, patients with Sturge–Weber syndrome do not have venous, lymphatic, or arterial anomalies in an extremity.
- Patients with Sturge–Weber syndrome are at increased risk for growth hormone deficiency and central hypothyroidism.

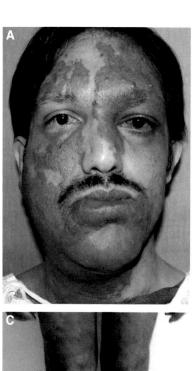

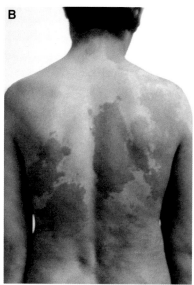

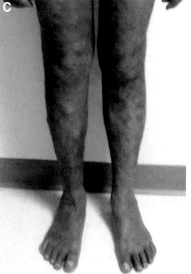

Fig. 13-6   Sturge-Weber syndrome. **A,** A 36-year-old man with glaucoma, seizures, and bilateral capillary malformations of the face involving the V_1, V_2, and V_3 trigeminal nerve distributions. Note pyogenic granulomas of his left forehead, and right lower lip overgrowth. **B** and **C,** The patient also has diffuse capillary malformations involving his trunk and lower extremities.

DIAGNOSIS

Imaging

• An MRI is obtained to rule out leptomeningeal vascular lesions, which are located ipsilateral to the facial capillary malformation and usually involve the parietal and occipital lobes.
• 75% of seizures occur during the first year of life; thus a screening MRI should be performed in infancy. If the MRI findings are negative, imaging should be repeated at 2 years of age, because false-negative findings can occur in young children, and some patients do not develop seizures until 3 years of age.
• Typical MRI findings of the leptomeningeal anomaly include enhancement, dilated deep draining veins, and an enlarged, enhancing choroid plexus.

Histopathology

• Histopathology is not specific for Sturge-Weber syndrome; diagnosis is made clinically by the presence of a facial capillary malformation with either eye or brain anomalies.
• Biopsy of the facial vascular malformation shows capillary malformation.

MANAGEMENT

• Any patient with a capillary malformation in an upper trigeminal nerve distribution should be screened for Sturge-Weber syndrome.
• If an abnormality is identified on a brain MRI, a neurologic consultation is obtained.
• Epilepsy is managed with seizure medications. Patients with seizures refractory to at least two medications are considered for resection of the epileptic focus.

- Patients undergo ophthalmologic evaluation to assess for choroidal anomalies and glaucoma every 6 months until 2 years of age, then yearly thereafter.
- Capillary malformation is managed similarly to nonsyndromic lesions:
  - Pulsed-dye laser treatment to lighten the malformation
  - Soft tissue and bony contouring if overgrowth occurs underneath the area of the stain

Selected References

Alomari AI. Characterization of a distinct syndrome that associates complex truncal overgrowth, vascular, and acral anomalies: a descriptive study of 18 cases of CLOVES syndrome. Clin Dysmorphol 18:1-7, 2009.

Cohen MM Jr. Proteus syndrome: an update. Am J Med Genet C Semin Med Genet 137C:38-52, 2005.

Greene AK, Kieran M, Burrows PE, Mulliken JB, Kasser J, Fishman SJ. Wilms tumor screening for Klippel–Trenaunay syndrome is unnecessary. Pediatrics 113:E326-E329, 2004.

Greene AK, Taber SF, Ball KL, Padwa BL, Mulliken JB. Sturge–Weber syndrome: frequency and morbidity of facial overgrowth. J Craniofac Surg 20:617-621, 2009.

Gupta A, Kozakewich H. Histopathology of vascular anomalies. Clin Plast Surg 38:31-44, 2011.

Kaplan RP, Wang JT, Amron DM, Kaplan L. Maffucci's syndrome: two case reports with a literature review. J Am Acad Dermatol 29:894-899, 1993.

Kulungowski AM, Fishman SJ. Management of combined vascular malformations. Clin Plast Surg 38:107-120, 2011.

Kurek KC, Luks VL, Ayturk UM, Alomari AI, Fishman SJ, Spencer SA, Mulliken JB, Bowen ME, Yamamoto GL, Kozakewich HP, Warman ML. Somatic mosaic activating mutations in PIK3CA cause CLOVES syndrome. Am J Hum Genet 90:1108-1115, 2012.

Lo W, Marchuk DA, Ball KL, Juhász C, Jordan LC, Ewen JB, Comi A. Updates and future horizons on the understanding, diagnosis, and treatment of Sturge-Weber syndrome brain involvement. Dev Med Child Neurol 54:214-223, 2012.

Pansuriya TC, van Eijk R, d'Adamo P, van Ruler MA, Kuijjer ML, Oosting J, Cleton-Jansen AM, van Oosterwijk JG, Verbeke SL, Meijer D, van Wezel T, Nord KH, Sangiorgi L, Toker B, Liegl-Atzwanger B, San-Julian M, Sciot R, Limaye N, Kindblom LG, Daugaard S, Godfraind C, Boon LM, Vikkula M, Kurek KC, Szuhai K, French PJ, Bovée JV. Somatic mosaic IDH1 and IDH2 mutations are associated with enchondroma and spindle cell hemangioma in Ollier disease and Maffucci syndrome. Nat Genet 43:1256-1261, 2011.

Revencu N, Boon LM, Mulliken JB, Enjolras O, Cordisco MR, Burrows PE, Clapuyt P, Hammer F, Dubois J, Baselga E, Brancati F, Carder R, Quintal JM, Dallapiccola B, Fischer G, Frieden IJ, Garzon M, Harper J, Johnson-Patel J, Labrèze C, Martorell L, Paltiel HJ, Pohl A, Prendiville J, Quere I, Siegel DH, Valente EM, Van Hagen A, Van Hest L, Vaux KK, Vicente A, Weibel L, Chitayat D, Vikkula M. Parkes Weber syndrome, vein of Galen aneurysmal malformation, and other fast-flow vascular anomalies are caused by RASA1 mutations. Hum Mutat 29:959-965, 2008.

Verdegaal SH, Bovée JV, Pansuriya TC, Grimer RJ, Ozger H, Jutte PC, San-Julian M, Biau DJ, van der Geest IC, Leithner A, Streitbürger A, Klenke FM, Gouin FG, Campanacci DA, Marec-Berard P, Hogendoorn PC, Brand R, Taminiau AH. Incidence, predictive factors, and prognosis of chondrosarcoma in patients with Ollier disease and Maffucci syndrome: an international multicenter study of 161 patients. Oncologist 16:1771-1779, 2011.

IV

Summary of Vascular Anomalies

CHAPTER 14

Diagnosis and Management

DIAGNOSIS OF VASCULAR ANOMALIES BY HISTORY

Major Types of Vascular Anomalies

- The field of vascular anomalies is confusing because different lesions often look similar, imprecise terminology is used, and many vascular anomalies exist. Eleven major types of vascular anomalies are listed with descriptions of over 40 subtypes of lesions.
- To simplify the diagnosis of a patient with a vascular anomaly, the health care provider should initially focus on the eight major categories of lesions (four tumors and four malformations) (Fig. 14-1). Approximately 98% of patients will have one of the four major types of vascular tumors (infantile hemangioma, congenital hemangioma, kaposiform hemangioendothelioma, or pyogenic granuloma) or one of the four major types of vascular malformations (capillary, lymphatic, venous, or arteriovenous).
- Only after the clinician identifies the major category of vascular anomaly should he or she consider a possible subtype of lesion.
- When examining a patient with a vascular anomaly, the health care provider must first establish an accurate diagnosis to offer correct treatment. The initial question to answer is: *Does the patient have a tumor or a malformation?* Once this is determined, the second question is: *Which of the four major types of tumors or malformations does the individual have?*
- An experienced clinician can discern the type of vascular anomaly by physical examination only. If this is not possible, the patient or family is asked about the patient's age when the lesion was first noted and the growth characteristics of the anomaly.

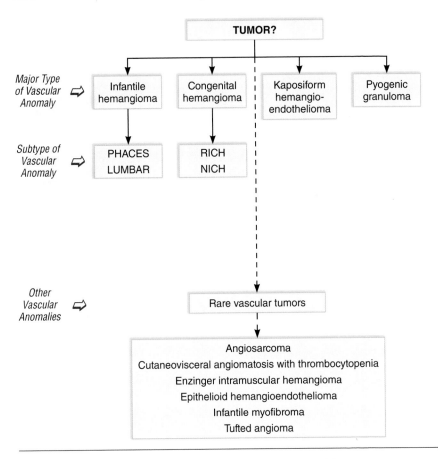

Fig. 14-1 Algorithm for diagnosing a vascular anomaly. When examining a patient with a vascular anomaly, the clinician should first determine whether the individual has a tumor or a malformation. Next, the lesion is assigned to one of the eight major types of vascular anomalies (four tumors and four malformations). Only after the major type of vascular anomaly is identified should the clinician determine whether the lesion is a subtype of one of the eight major vascular anomalies. Rare vascular tumors and malformation overgrowth syndromes compose 2% or less of vascular anomalies and should only be considered after ruling out the common vascular anomalies and subtypes. (*PHACES,* Posterior fossa brain malformation, hemangioma, arterial cerebrovascular anomalies, coarctation of the aorta and cardiac defects, eye/endocrine abnormalities, sternal clefting/supraumbilical raphe; *LUMBAR,* lower body infantile hemangioma, urogenital anomalies/ulceration, myelopathy, bony

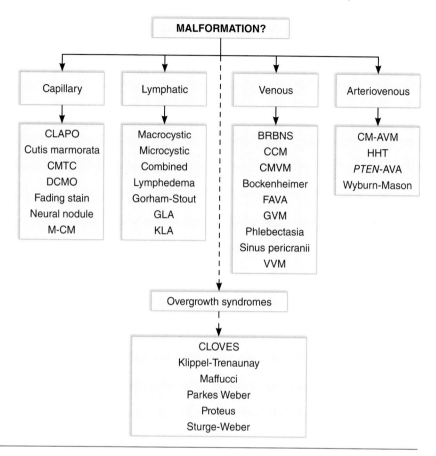

deformities, anorectal malformations/arterial anomalies, and renal anomalies; *RICH*, rapidly involuting congenital hemangioma; *NICH*, noninvoluting congenital hemangioma; *CLAPO*, capillary malformation of the lower lip, lymphatic malformation of the face and neck, asymmetry, and partial/generalized overgrowth; *CMTC*, cutis marmorata telangiectatica congenita; *DCMO*, diffuse capillary malformation with overgrowth; *M-CM*, macrocephaly–capillary malformation; *GLA*, generalized lymphatic anomaly; *KLA*, kaposiform lymphangiomatosis; *BRBNS*, blue rubber bleb nevus syndrome; *CCM*, cerebral cavernous malformation; *CMVM*, cutaneomucosal venous malformation; *FAVA*, fibroadipose vascular anomaly; *GVM*, glomuvenous malformation; *VVM*, verrucous venous malformation; *CM-AVM*, capillary malformation–arteriovenous malformation; *HHT*, hereditary hemorrhagic telangiectasia; *PTEN-AVA*, PTEN-associated vascular anomaly.)

Differentiating Vascular Anomalies Based on Age of Onset

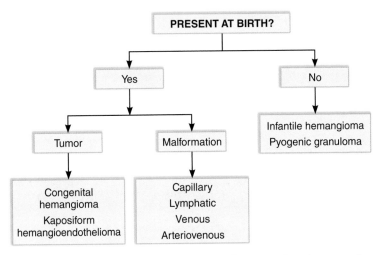

Fig. 14-2   Algorithm for diagnosing a vascular anomaly using age of onset.

- If the diagnosis of a vascular anomaly is not obvious on physical examination, the first question to ask is: *When did you first notice the lesion?* It is most important to discern whether the vascular anomaly was present at birth, because this information can be used to differentiate lesions (Fig. 14-2).
- It is critical to differentiate an infantile hemangioma, which is very common, from other vascular anomalies. Infantile hemangioma is often noted 1 or 2 weeks after birth, but a cutaneous discoloration may exist at birth. Parents often state that the infantile hemangioma was present "at birth," but if they are asked if the lesion was there *immediately after delivery,* they will respond that it was not noticed at that time.

- If a vascular anomaly is present at birth, then possible tumors include congenital hemangioma or kaposiform hemangioendothelioma.
- All malformations are present at birth (although they may not be appreciated until a later time): capillary, lymphatic, venous, and arteriovenous.
- If the vascular anomaly was not recognized at birth, potential tumors include infantile hemangioma or pyogenic granuloma.
- Infantile hemangioma may be first noted as late as 4 months of age if it is located subcutaneously. Pyogenic granuloma rarely occurs during the first year of life.
- Although malformations are present at birth, they may not be noted until later in life, after they have slowly enlarged or become symptomatic. Consequently, *if a vascular anomaly is not recognized at birth, it does not rule out a vascular malformation.*

Differentiating Vascular Anomalies Based on Postnatal Growth

- After determining whether the vascular anomaly was present at birth, patients or families are asked: *After you discovered the lesion, did it increase, decrease, or stay the same size?*
- Rapid postnatal growth can occur with two major types of tumors. Infantile hemangioma will have significant growth over the first several weeks of life, which is unique to this tumor. Pyogenic granuloma usually enlarges rapidly after it is first noted.
- Slow postnatal growth may occur with one major type of tumor and all malformations. Kaposiform hemangioendothelioma (a tumor) can expand during the first 2 years of life. Capillary, lymphatic, venous, and arteriovenous malformations usually enlarge over the course of the patient's lifetime.

- No postnatal growth can occur with one major type of tumor and all malformations. Congenital hemangioma (a tumor) does not enlarge postnatally. Capillary, lymphatic, venous, and arteriovenous malformations may remain stable long-term.
- Postnatal regression occurs with two major types of tumors only. Infantile hemangioma becomes smaller beginning at approximately 12 months of age and continues to shrink until 3 to 4 years of age. Rapidly involuting congenital hemangioma regresses immediately after birth and has completed involution by 14 months of age.

Minor Types of Vascular Anomalies

- When diagnosing a patient with a vascular anomaly, the clinician should first determine whether the lesion is a tumor or a malformation. Next, he or she will decide which of the eight major types of vascular anomalies categories the lesion belongs to: tumors (infantile hemangioma, congenital hemangioma, kaposiform hemangioendothelioma, or pyogenic granuloma) or malformations (capillary, lymphatic, venous, or arteriovenous) (see Fig. 14-1).
- Only after the clinician has determined which of the eight major categories of vascular anomalies the lesion fits into should he or she attempt to identify the particular subtype of lesion (for example, a macrocystic lymphatic malformation or glomuvenous malformation). There are more than 40 subtypes of vascular anomalies, and with experience, identifying the specific subtype becomes easier.
- If the clinician is able to adequately diagnose the patient with one of the eight major types of vascular anomalies, it is likely the patient will be treated correctly. However, many subtypes are managed differently. For example, macrocystic lymphatic malformations are treated with sclerotherapy, whereas microcystic lesions are managed primarily by resection.
- Only 1% or 2% of vascular anomalies do not fit into the eight major categories of lesions. These individuals will have either a

rare vascular tumor or a vascular malformation overgrowth syndrome. Rare tumors or overgrowth syndromes should be considered only after determining that the patient does not have one of the more common types of vascular anomalies.

DIAGNOSIS OF VASCULAR ANOMALIES BY PHYSICAL EXAMINATION

Differentiating Vascular Anomalies by Appearance

- Infantile hemangioma is red, although it can appear bluish or have no overlying skin changes if it is located beneath the skin.
- Congenital hemangioma is more purple than infantile hemangioma, has a surrounding pale halo, and contains large telangiectasias.
- Kaposiform hemangioendothelioma is reddish-purple.
- Pyogenic granuloma is red and usually has a stalk.
- Capillary malformation is pink during early childhood and becomes purple as the patient ages.
- Venous malformation is blue, but if located beneath the integument, it may not have overlying skin discoloration. Venous malformation can be confirmed: it is the only vascular anomaly that significantly enlarges if placed in a dependent position.
- Lymphatic malformation can appear pink or blue and may contain cutaneous red vesicles. If it is located beneath the skin, the overlying integument may appear normal.
- Arteriovenous malformation can appear pink or red.

Differentiating Vascular Anomalies by Size

- Infantile hemangioma can range from 1 mm in diameter to a diffuse lesion involving a large anatomic area.
- Congenital hemangioma is well defined and is typically larger than an infantile hemangioma (the average diameter is 5 cm).
- Kaposiform hemangioendothelioma is typically diffuse and large (greater than 5 cm).

- Pyogenic granuloma is solitary and small (the average diameter is 6.5 mm).
- Capillary malformation, lymphatic malformation, venous malformation, and arteriovenous malformation can range from small, localized lesions to diffuse malformations involving large anatomic areas.

Differentiating Vascular Anomalies by Location

- Infantile hemangioma and pyogenic granuloma most commonly involve the head or neck, but can affect any cutaneous site.
- Congenital hemangioma affects the limbs (45%), head or neck (43%), or trunk (12%).
- Kaposiform hemangioendothelioma involves the head or neck (40%), trunk (30%), or extremity (30%).
- Capillary malformation is most commonly located on the head or neck, but it can affect any area of integument.
- Lymphatic malformation most frequently affects the neck or axilla, but it can be located throughout the body.
- Venous malformation is more likely than other vascular malformations to involve muscle, but it can be located in almost any anatomic location.
- Arteriovenous malformation more commonly affects the head or neck, but it can involve the trunk or extremities as well.

Differentiating Vascular Anomalies by Symptoms

- Infantile hemangioma may ulcerate during infancy (16%), and it rarely bleeds.
- Congenital hemangioma ulcerates less often than infantile hemangioma and does not bleed.
- Kaposiform hemangioendothelioma typically causes pain and Kasabach–Merritt phenomenon: thrombocytopenia (platelet count below 25,000/mm^3), petechiae, and bleeding.
- Pyogenic granuloma often ulcerates and usually bleeds.
- Capillary malformation is usually asymptomatic.

- Lymphatic malformation can cause cutaneous leaking of lymph fluid, infection, intralesional bleeding, and pain.
- Venous malformation can be painful because of phlebothrombosis.
- Arteriovenous malformations can ulcerate and bleed.

Differentiating Vascular Anomalies Based on Blood Flow

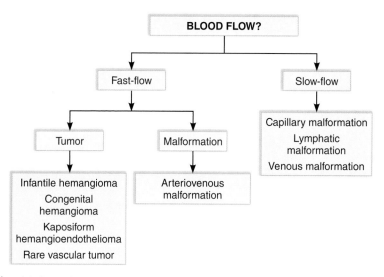

Fig. 14-3   Algorithm for diagnosing a vascular anomaly by evaluation of blood flow.

- Most vascular anomalies can be diagnosed by their appearance and history.
- If the clinician is unable to diagnosis the type of vascular anomaly by its history and appearance, a handheld Doppler probe is used to audibly assess the blood flow in the lesion (Fig. 14-3). The nonaffected contralateral area is assessed first to obtain a baseline signal, which is then compared with the blood flow in the vascular anomaly.

- If fast-flow is present, the lesion is either a tumor or arteriovenous malformation.
- If slow-flow is found, the anomaly is either a capillary, lymphatic, or venous malformation.

DIAGNOSIS OF VASCULAR ANOMALIES BY IMAGING

- More than 90% of vascular anomalies can be diagnosed by history and physical examination if the clinician uses the correct terminology, recognizes the clinical appearance of the lesion, and can differentiate anomalies based on age of onset and blood flow.
- Approximately 10% of vascular anomalies cannot be diagnosed by history and physical examination; thus imaging is required. Generally, ultrasonography is the first study used to aid the diagnosis of a vascular anomaly. If the type of lesion remains equivocal following ultrasound, an MRI is performed. Pyogenic granuloma and capillary malformation are not diagnosed by imaging.
- A proliferating infantile hemangioma and congenital hemangioma show fast-flow, shunting, and a parenchymal mass.
- Kaposiform hemangioendothelioma has fast-flow and shunting. The tumor invades adjacent tissues, and lymphatic involvement causes subcutaneous fat stranding.
- Lymphatic malformation exhibits macrocysts or microcysts. After a contrast medium is administered, macrocystic lesions show only enhancement of the wall. Compared with venous malformations, lymphatic malformations are less well defined and are more likely to infiltrate through tissue planes.
- Venous malformation demonstrates slow-flow and phleboliths. Lesions show diffuse, heterogeneous enhancement after contrast administration (unlike lymphatic malformation). Venous malformations are typically well circumscribed, lobulated, and can be isolated to an anatomic structure (usually muscle).
- Arteriovenous malformation exhibits hypervascularity, with fast-flow and shunting. Unlike hemangioma, a parenchymal mass is

not present. Dilated feeding arteries or draining veins, enhancement, and flow-voids are present. Angiography shows feeding arterial vessels, early filling of draining veins, and a nidus.

DIAGNOSIS OF VASCULAR ANOMALIES BY HISTOPATHOLOGY

- Only 1% of vascular anomalies require histopathologic evaluation for diagnosis. Rarely, the type of lesion remains unclear even after analysis.
- Infantile hemangioma uniquely expresses GLUT1.
- Congenital hemangioma can be differentiated from infantile hemangioma because it does not immunostain for GLUT1.
- Kaposiform hemangioendothelioma is an infiltrative lesion with lobules containing round or spindled endothelial cells and pericytes (the tumor can have a glomeruloid appearance). Hemosiderin-filled slit-like vascular spaces are present with red blood cell fragments and dilated lymphatics.
- Pyogenic granuloma is a polypoid dermal lesion with lobules of thin-walled capillaries with plump endothelial cells. Lesions usually involve the reticular dermis. The epithelium is atrophic, often ulcerated, and may have granulation tissue as well as lateral collarettes.
- Capillary malformation has a papillary dermis that contains dilated capillaries with thin walls and narrow lumens. As the child ages, the vessel size and density increase.
- Lymphatic malformations have small, thin-walled lymphatic channels with flat endothelial cells without smooth muscle. Lymphatic channels can contain eosinophilic protein-rich fluid with lymphocytes, macrophages, red blood cells, and/or hemosiderin. Because lymphatic malformations express lymphatic markers (D240, LYVE1, PROX1), they can be differentiated from other vascular anomalies immunohistochemically.
- Venous malformations exhibit veins that are irregular, lined by flat endothelium, and have a paucity of smooth muscle cells.

Thrombi are common in vessel lumens, and papillary endothelial hyperplasia may be present.
- Arteriovenous malformations show large, tortuous arteries with thick-walled veins. Arteries may have disrupted internal elastic lamina, and veins contain thickened muscular walls that become fibrotic.

MANAGEMENT OF VASCULAR ANOMALIES

- Treatment of a vascular anomaly should never be initiated until a definitive diagnosis has been established. The type of lesion is determined by history and physical examination, but imaging and/or histopathology may be necessary. Many types of treatments exist for vascular anomalies, which can be confusing to the clinician (for example, corticosteroid injection, embolization, excision, laser, prednisolone, propranolol, radiofrequency ablation, sclerotherapy, sirolimus, and vincristine).
- An infantile hemangioma is usually observed during the proliferating phase (90%). Localized problematic lesions are treated with corticosteroid injection. Tumors that are too large to inject are managed with systemic pharmacotherapy (either prednisolone or propranolol). Residual deformities can be treated with pulsed-dye laser or operative intervention in early childhood.
- A congenital hemangioma is observed. Operative intervention to correct a residual deformity is considered in early childhood.
- Kaposiform hemangioendothelioma is treated with vincristine to control Kasabach-Merritt phenomenon and/or to reduce fibrosis and chronic pain. Sirolimus has recently been used to treat this tumor.
- A pyogenic granuloma is resected to improve the deformity as well as to prevent ulceration and bleeding.
- A capillary malformation is managed with pulsed-dye laser to lighten the stain. Overgrowth underneath the malformation is treated by resection.

- A lymphatic malformation is managed by sclerotherapy if it is macrocystic. Resection is reserved for microcystic lesions or for macrocystic lymphatic malformations that remain symptomatic following sclerotherapy. Cutaneous or intraoral vesicles can be treated with carbon dioxide laser or radiofrequency ablation, respectively.
- Venous malformation is managed by sclerotherapy. Small lesions or those that are symptomatic after sclerotherapy are resected.
- Arteriovenous malformation is treated with embolization and/ or excision.

CONCLUSIONS

- Clinicians managing patients with vascular anomalies must use standardized terminology to ensure that the patient is treated correctly.
- Approximately 90% of vascular anomalies should be diagnosed by history and physical examination, about 99% after imaging, and close to 100% if histopathology is required.
- Treatment of a vascular anomaly is not considered until the diagnosis is confirmed.
- An experienced physician can manage most vascular anomalies independently. However, many lesions require interdisciplinary care and should be referred to a vascular anomalies center.
- Although vascular tumors are at least 10 times more common than vascular malformations, vascular malformations are generally more problematic, and therefore two thirds of patients managed in a vascular anomalies center are treated for vascular malformations.
- As the pathophysiology of different vascular anomalies continues to be elucidated (Table 14-1), improved therapeutic strategies will be developed.
- If the clinician initially focuses on the eight major types of vascular anomalies, he or she will be able to manage approximately 95% of patients correctly (Table 14-2).

Table 14-1   *Vascular Anomalies With Known Mutations*

CONDITION

Venous Malformations

Sporadic venous malformation (VM)
Glomuvenous malformation (GVM)
Cutaneomucosal venous malformation (VMCM)
Cerebral cavernous malformation (CCM1, CCM2, CCM3)

Lymphatic Malformations

Familial congenital primary lymphedema (Milroy)
Lymphedema-distichiasis
Lymphedema-hypotrichosis-telangiectasia
Hennekam syndrome

Arteriovenous Malformations

Capillary malformation–arteriovenous malformation
Hereditary hemorrhagic telangiectasia (HHT1, HHT2)
Hereditary hemorrhagic telangiectasia-juvenile polyposis
PTEN-associated vascular anomaly

Vascular Malformation Syndromes

CLOVES
Klippel-Trenaunay
Maffucci
Parkes Weber
Proteus

MUTATED GENE	MODE OF INHERITANCE
TIE2 (40% to 50%)	Somatic
Glomulin	Dominant
TIE2	Dominant
KRIT1/malcavernin/ PDCD10	Dominant
VEGFR3	Dominant/recessive
FOXC2	Dominant
SOX18	Dominant/recessive
CCBE1	Dominant/recessive
RASA1	Dominant
ENG/ACVRL1	Dominant
SMAD4	Dominant
PTEN	Dominant
PIK3CA	Somatic
PIK3CA	Somatic
IDH1/IDH2	Somatic
RASA1	Dominant
AKT1	Somatic

Table 14-2   *Summary of the Eight Major Types of Vascular Anomalies*

VASCULAR TUMORS

Type	Diagnosis	Management
Infantile hemangioma	History Physical examination Ultrasound	Observation Corticosteroid injection Prednisolone Propranolol Resection
Congenital hemangioma	History Physical examination	Observation Resection
Kaposiform hemangio- endothelioma	History Physical examination MRI Histopathology	Vincristine Sirolimus
Pyogenic granuloma	History Physical examination	Resection

VASCULAR MALFORMATIONS		
Type	**Diagnosis**	**Management**
Capillary malformation	History Physical examination	Observation Laser Resection
Lymphatic malformation	History Physical examination Ultrasound MRI	Observation Sclerotherapy Resection
Venous malformation	History Physical examination Ultrasound MRI	Observation Sclerotherapy Resection
Arteriovenous malformation	History Physical examination Ultrasound MRI Angiogram	Observation Embolization Resection

INDEX